Advance Praise

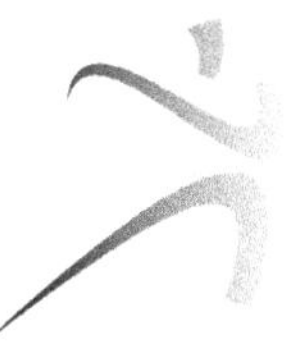

Mr. Prosper's book is a simple roadmap to achieving your personal fitness goals. For anyone out there, be it the hardcore fitness fanatic or the individual new to the fitness scene, this book is the definitive blueprint to a rock hard body. This book is a must have in the collection for fitness gurus, fighters and the average Joe's everywhere.

– DAVID D'ANTONIO, Owner of (C.U.T.S.,) Critical Urban Tactical Strategies, *Philadelphia, Pennsylvania*

"Urgent necessity prompts many to do things."–*Miguel de Cervantes*

Charles is a (Master Motivator) who lives by example. In this book he demonstrates his unique ability to reach out to each and every individual regardless of age or handicap, to push beyond their own expectations for a healthier self. After reading this book, you won't even think about quitting your routine or getting out of shape!

– ANDY CURTISS, Certified Sports Trainer and Nutritionist, *U.S.A.*

Don't be fooled by the title! This is a great nutrition and exercise program that is for both men and women of all age groups. Complete and in plain English!

– DENISE KENNY, black belt Kyokushin Kai Karate, *Moncton, New Brunswick Canada*

How To Get Fit Fast At Any Age is more then just your average fitness book. It not only inspires you to get fit physically but inspires you spiritually and mentally as well. Your perception and attitude towards fitness will change exponentially after you have read this book.

– NORM BETTENCOURT, author, *Secrets of Street Fighting*, *Vancouver, B.C. Canada*

Charles, after reading your book, I truly believe you have something here. The principles are simple, explicit and thorough. The material dispels myths about dieting and explains why diets dont work. It talks about thinking in terms of changing my behaviors, understanding what food is and does. You've discussed goal setting, and how to eat clean. Something I have forgotten. And you have provided me with a plan of action that is simple enough to keep me on target. Charles, the work you've have done here is nothing less than "masterful".

– Andrew Campbell, *Inland Empire, California*

Wow! You have so much information in there, and it's so easy to follow. I like all your explanations and the info on nutrition and eating. Well done - a fantastic book!

– John Byrne, *Newport, Isle of Wight, United Kingdom*

"Necessity is the mother of taking chances."*–*Mark Twain

How To Get Fit Fast At Any Age is an inspirational guide of the physical, mental, and emotional benefits of exercise. .... And as this book asserts, it's never too late to get fit. It is no longer how old you are, but how old you want to be. It is easy to read and easy to follow. The well laid out exercise program clearly explains and helps the fitness pros as well as the first-timers devise their own regimens and become healthier in all areas of life. Great book, Charles!

– Roger Boggs, Owner, Goshin Karate & Judo Academy, *Scottsdale, Arizona*

A wonderful guide and mentor that is capable of being understood and implemented by the ordinary man in the street as well as the experts in fitness and health - changing one's life for the better!

– Buddy Govender, Chief Instructor, Oju Ryu Okinawa Karate, *Durban, South Africa*

The book is overloaded with lots of information. Its content is actually good enough for use as a textbook for college courses or a certificated program.

– Randy Li, *Overland Park, Kansas*

HOW TO GET FIT FAST AT ANY AGE

"It is no longer how old you are but how old you want to be"

Charles Prosper

First Edition

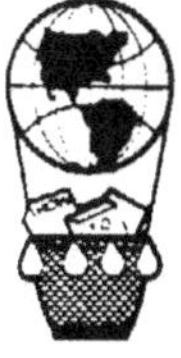

Global Publishing Company • Los Angeles, California

HOW TO GET FIT FAST AT ANY AGE

"It is no longer how old you are but how old you want to be"

by Charles Prosper

LEGAL DISCLAIMER:

Global Publishing Company takes no legal responsibility for any physical injury or harm you may sustain if you improperly use the information, diet or exercises contained in How To Get Fit Fast At Any Age. You must consult with your doctor before starting any physical routine or exercise program to prevent any physical injuries, especially if you are over 40 or 50 years old.

Book layout design and cover design by Charles Prosper

LIBRARY OF CONGRESS CATALOG CARD DATA

ISBN–13 978-0-943845-06-7

PRINTED IN THE UNITED STATES OF AMERICA

12 11 10 9 8 7 6 5 4 3 2 1

For my dear daughter, Luzemily, who has always loved me through thick and thin, fat and slim

CONTENTS

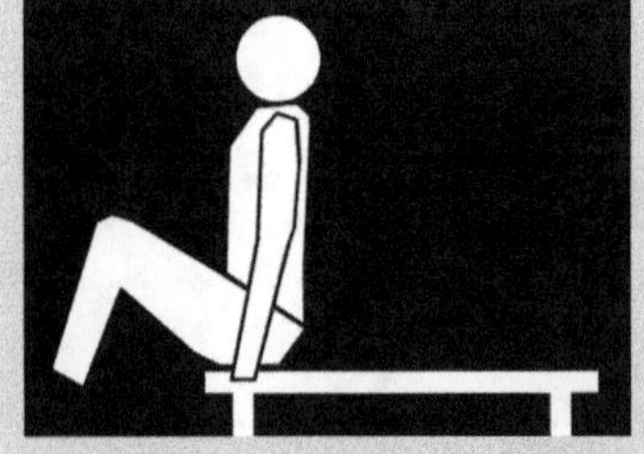
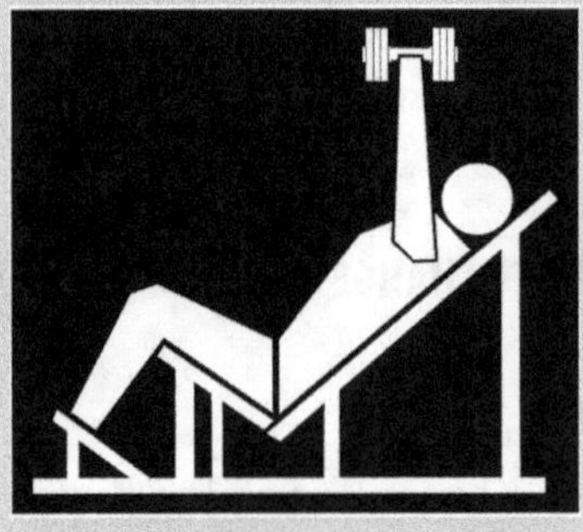
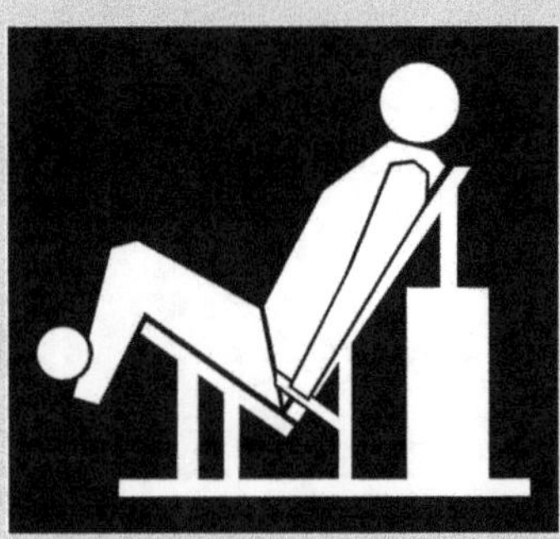
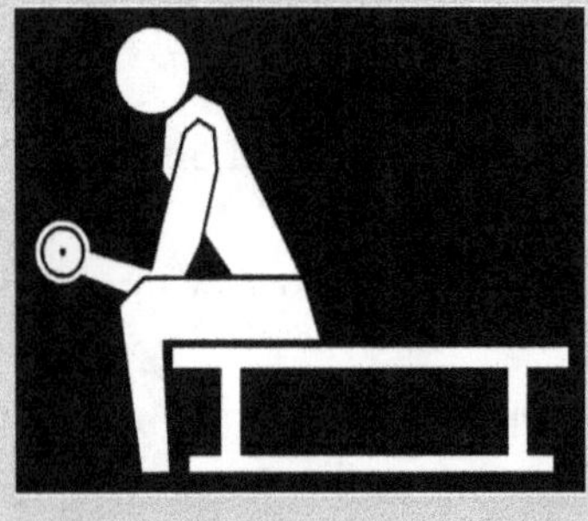

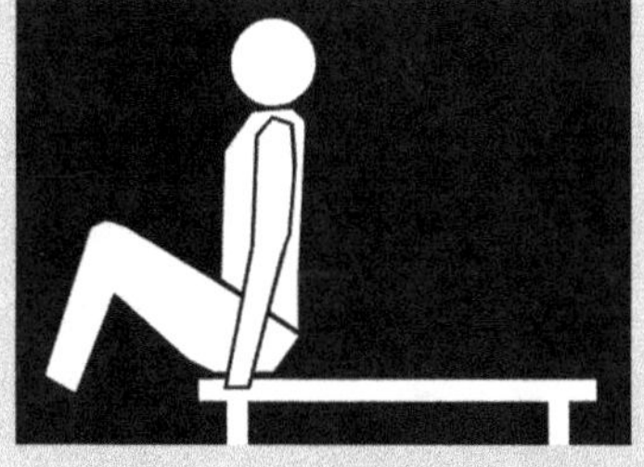
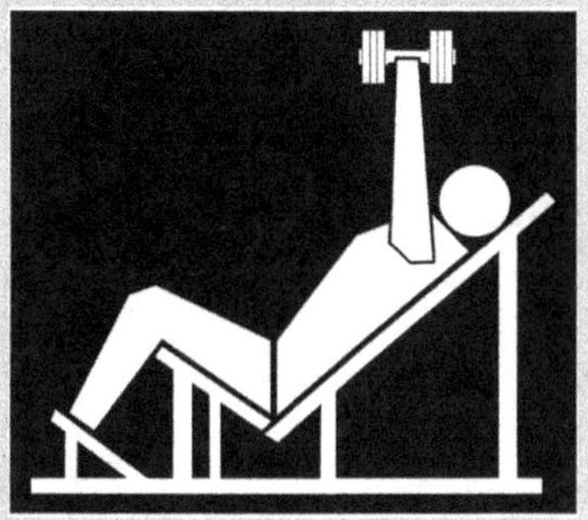
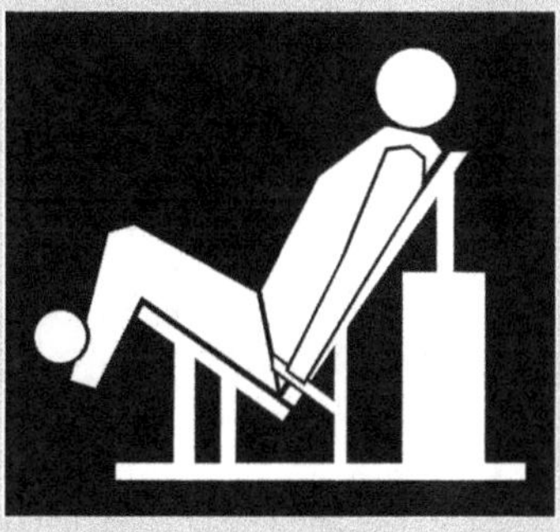
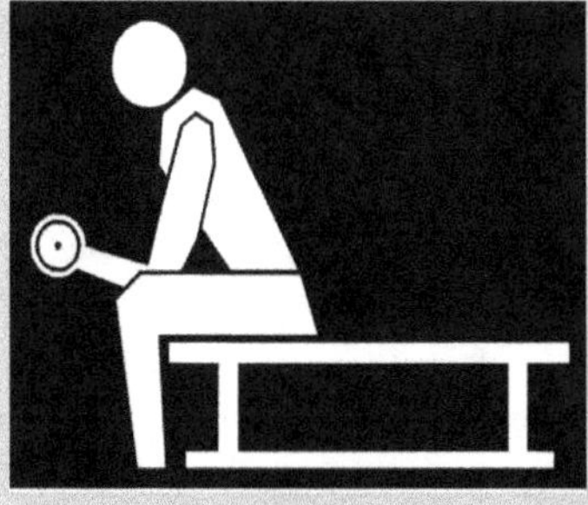

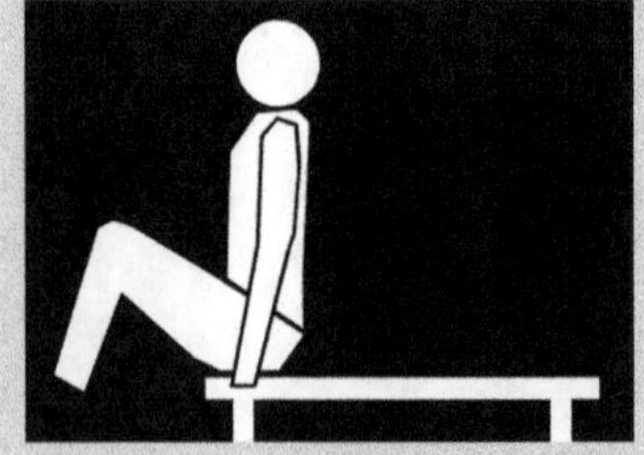
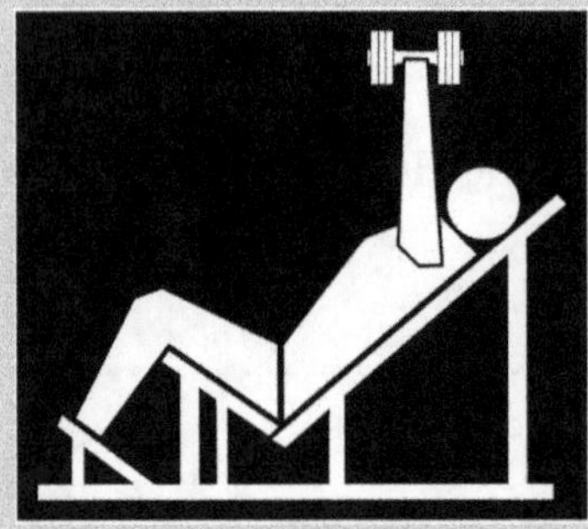
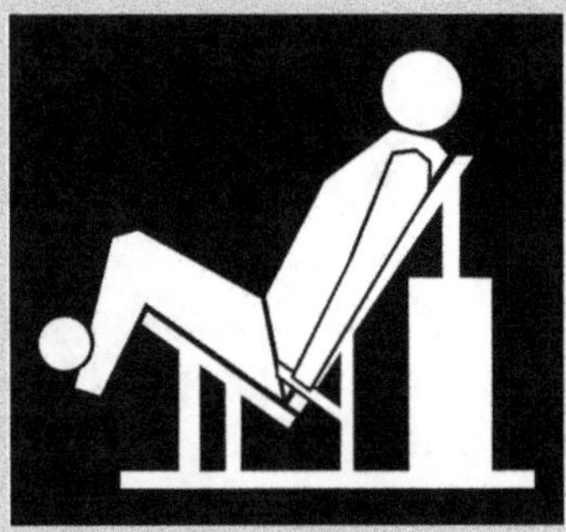
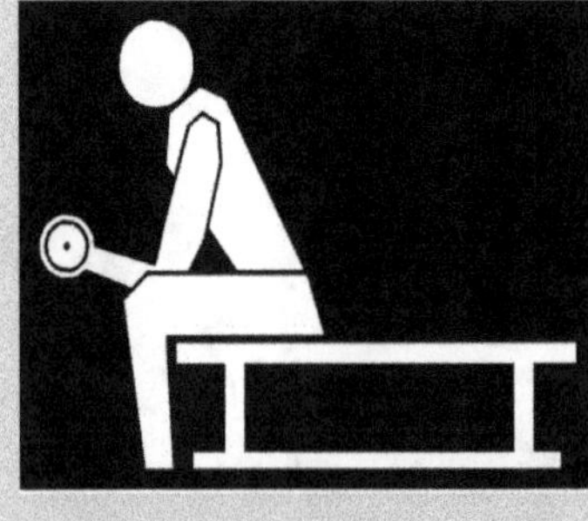

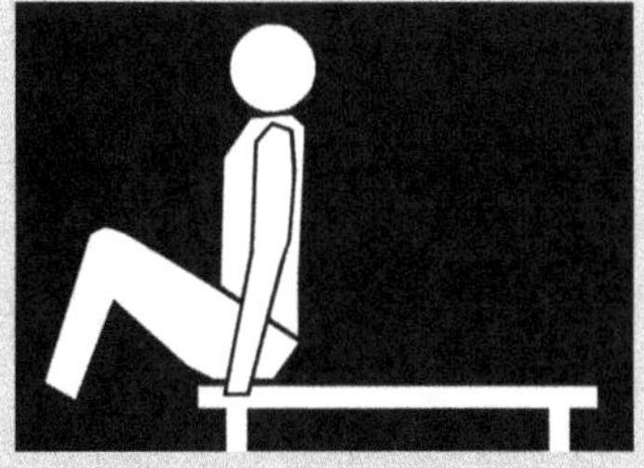
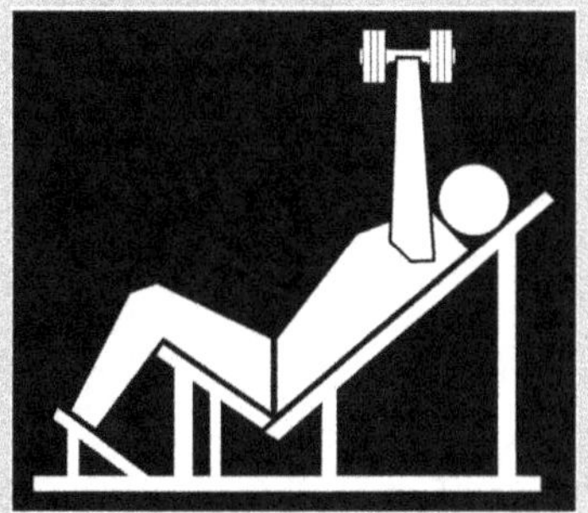
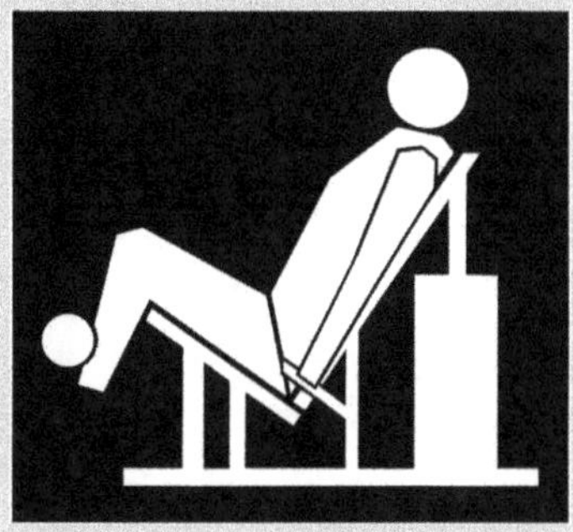
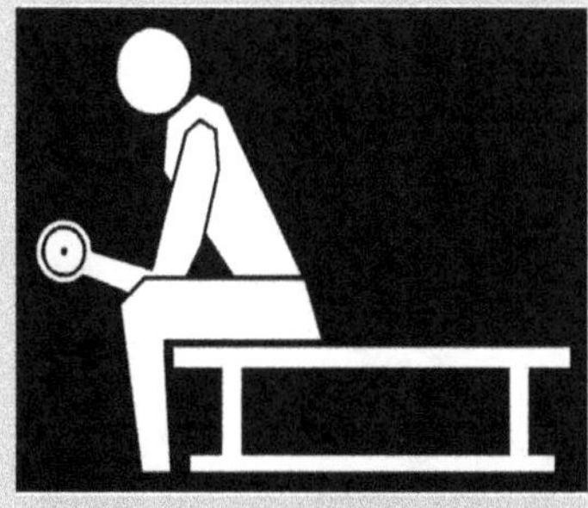

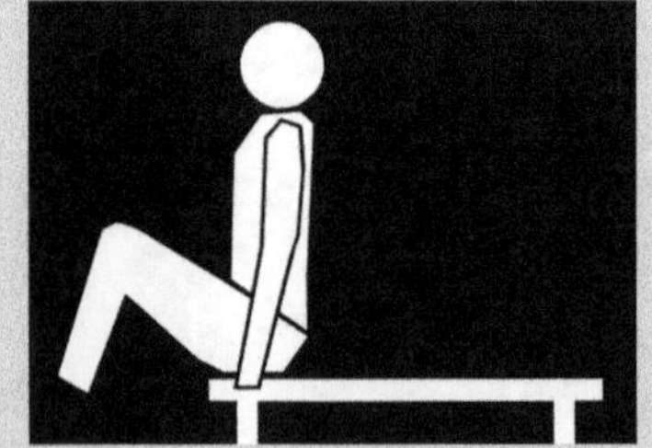

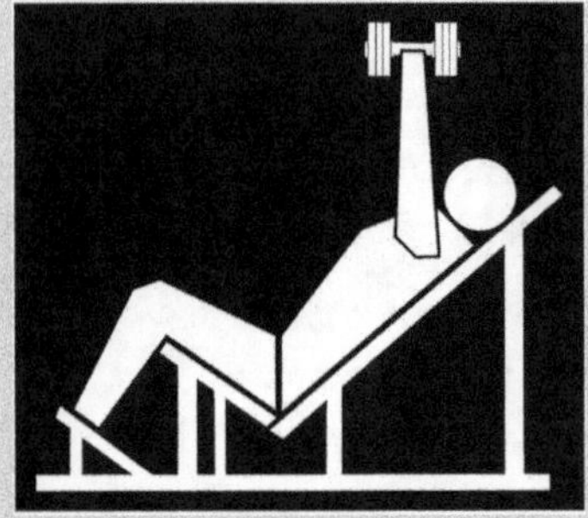

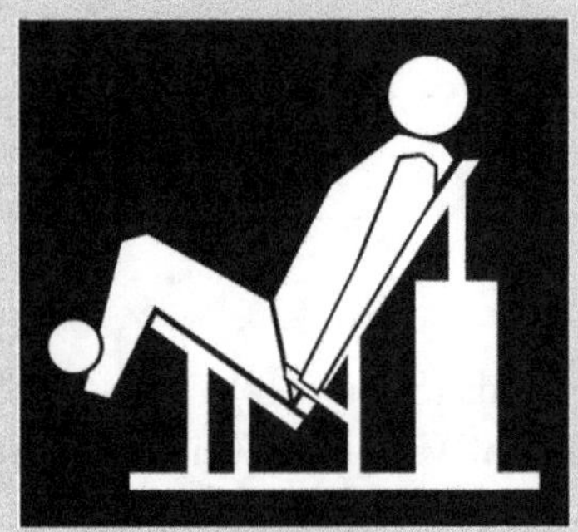

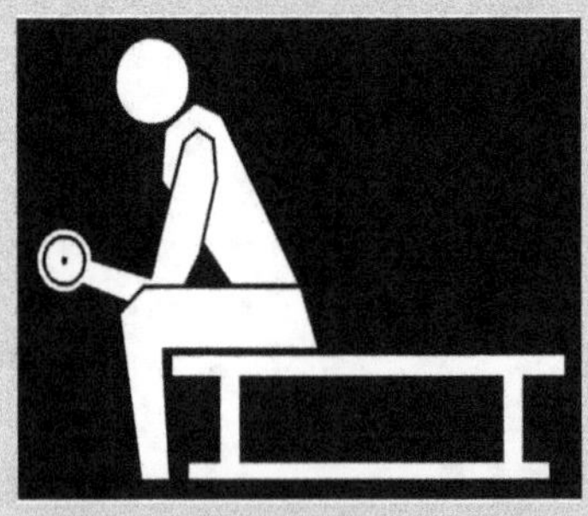

ACKNOWLEDGMENTS

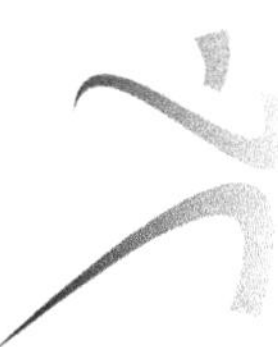

No great work is accomplished alone. I want to sincerely thank my good friend **Denise Brideau Kenny** for her sharp and eagle eye in catching and correcting the plethora of my glitches and misspellings in the rough draft of the book. Denise, with all of your love and talent, you have blessed my book and have made it holy.

Did you notice the great color shots on the back cover and all of the great outdoor black and white shots of me demonstrating the exercises in the book? This marvelous job of photography was done by none other than my beautiful 11-year old daughter, **Luzemily**.

And I would indeed be remiss in not to acknowledge the book cover's beautiful color photography by **Frank Aguilera** of *Aguilera Video Productions,* Bell, California.

"Faith is the currency of miracles."–Charles Prosper

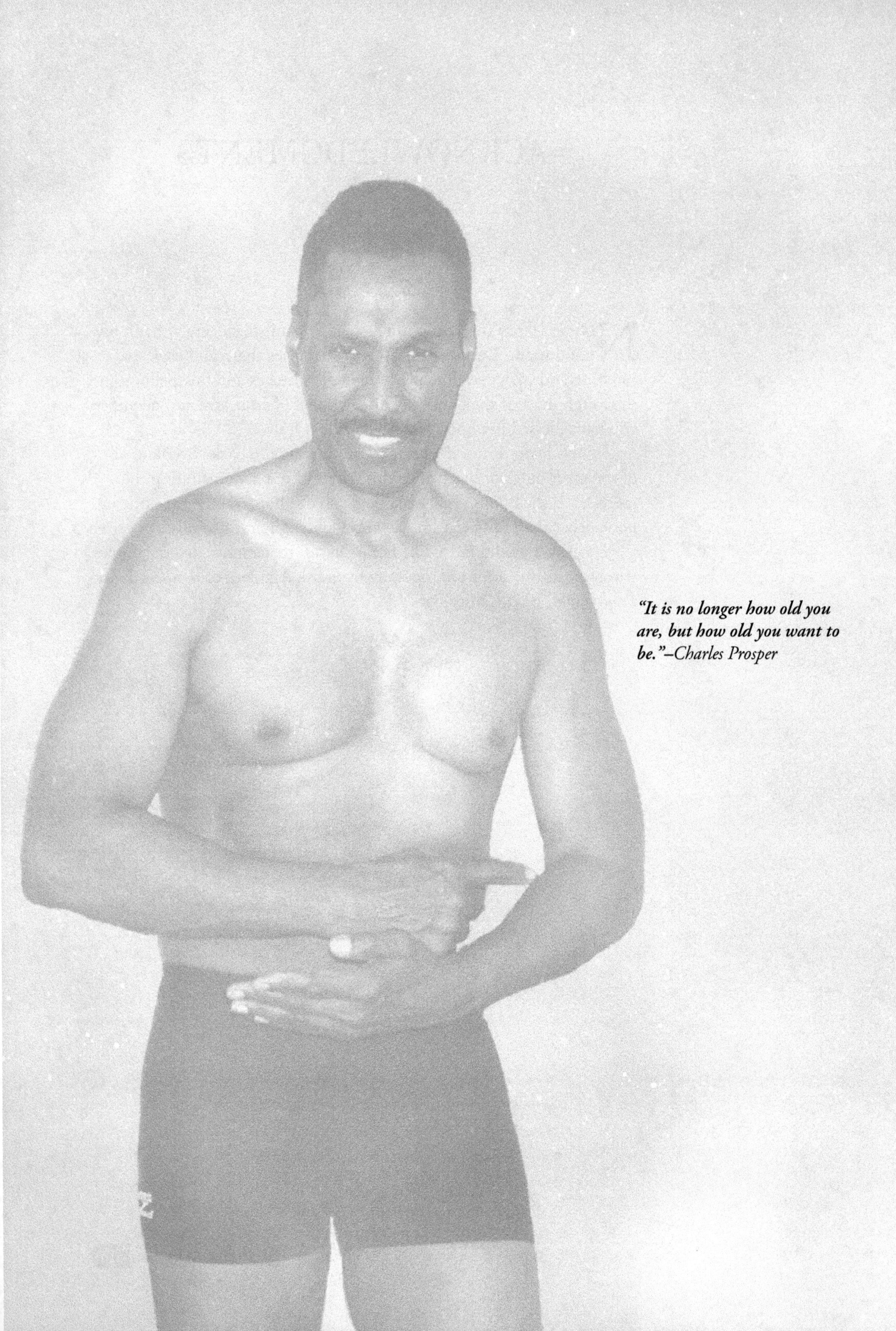

"It is no longer how old you are, but how old you want to be."–Charles Prosper

INTRODUCTION

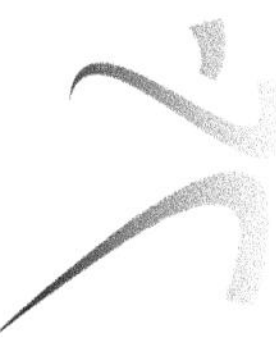

Whatever made you pick up this book, I want to commend you. You just can't imagine what an important step that you have taken. You may not know me personally, but I feel that we know each other in the sense that we are kindred spirits who seek the best that we can be in body, mind and spirit. In this work, I will primarily address the body aspect of the triad of your existence, and I will particularly target those who believe that it is too late for them to be in the best shape of their lives. If you are 30, 40, 50, 60 or 70, and you want a safe and sure way to dip into the fountain of youth, stay with me, a miracle in your life is about to happen – *in a matter of as little as just 12 weeks.* Just give me 12 weeks of a chance, follow my instructions to the "T", and you will not recognize yourself when you step in front of the mirror.

"It's not important that you know everything–just the important things."–Miguel de Unamuno

It Is No Longer How Old You Are, But How Old You Want To Be

This is fitness program that I will lay out for you, will establish a new paradigm for age. That new paradigm quite simply put is "It is no longer how old you are, but how old you want to be." Look, none of us can stop chronological time, this is just out of our control. And really, who cares about chronological time, if I can place your tired 50-year old body in a new one of the looks and energy level of a 30-year old, who cares about the number of candles on a cake.

I understand and accept that our modern-day society is full of what I call "age bigots". What I mean by that is that once you reach a certain age, people in general will make certain assumptions about you, that is, you can no longer do this, or you no longer can do that, and so on and so forth. I rarely reveal my age, but if you saw me in person, I guarantee that you would not judge me more that 48 years or so, yet I am over fifty – fit and sexy as ever! This is not by luck and this is not by chance. This is by design. I have been able to turn back the clock and *slow* down the aging process enormously, *and you will too!* The keys to the fountain of youth lay awaiting in your hands in this book. No matter what anyone has to say about it in preference for any other system of weight loss, body sculpting and fitness, what I will show you in these pages has one distinct advantage – *it works!*

I will show you in this book how to get fit fast over thirty, forty, fifty, sixty or seventy. You will learn that *you still got it*, be you male or female. You will learn how to transform your body, no matter what shape it is, into a sleek and sexy body work of art in only 3 months. Yes, that is only 12 weeks to totally change your life forever.

You will discover how easy it is to:

- **Reach your ideal weight in as little as 12 weeks!**
  I am not asking much of you. I am only asking that you give this program a fair try of only 3 months, and I guarantee that you will never be the same. Your whole outlook and attitude for life will change for the better. You will look good, feel good and live good.

- **Eat 5 times a day and still lose weight!**
  Yes, you read right. You will learn how to eat more meals, though smaller and well-planned nutrition-wise, and still be able to lose pounds of fat that will just dissolve and melt off your body revealing a leaner, sexier you - at *<u>any</u>* age!

"There is no such thing as good luck or bad luck–only how you think of yourself."– *Luzemily Prosper (10-years old)*

- **Take unwanted fat off and <u>keep</u> it off!**
  Any crash diet can cause you to lose weight, but as all diets go, after you stop the madness, your body realizes that this temporary sacrifice is over, it will be more than happy to help you to make up for lost time by packing all of those quickly lost pounds back on you, and a little extra just to be ready for the next time. Bottom line. Diets don't work. Diets have never worked, will never work, and because of their nature, they are designed unintentionally to never work. Why? Because the definition of diet is a *temporary* deviation from normal, healthy eating for the purpose of quick weight loss. What I teach you here is not a diet, but a new lifestyle of clean, healthy eating, in the right portions and with a delightful variety of satisfying foods. No hunger fasts here – just good clean eating for life.

- **Become firm, tone and muscular at *<u>any</u>* age**
  One of the most impressively fit gentlemen I have ever met in my life was David, a young man of 70 years young. I met him about 18 years ago while visiting Gold's Gym of Venice, California. I was totally blown away! He had the body of a slim and fit 35-year old man at the most. I commended him on his excellent shape, and he replied: "Thanks, and it keeps

your sex drive up." Though I was younger then, this was the first time that I began to think of age in a totally different and more positive way.

- **Lower your cholesterol and improve your blood pressure**
  I can't even count the number of people whom I have met that have been able to lower their blood serum cholesterol as well as improve their blood pressure following the regimen of clean eating and progressive weight resistance that I will outline for you.

- **Sleep better at night**
  One of many positive things that you will notice is that you will begin to sleep like a baby. The quality of your sleep will improve. You will find yourself waking up, more and more, each day feeling well-rested, energized and ready to take on the day.

- **Increase your sex drive**
  Progressive weight resistance coupled with clean, health eating is nature's natural Viagra. Testosterone levels rise, and you know what that means! Party-time with your clothes off. Sex lives of both men and women will get better simply because you will feel like doing it more. Your energy level, in time, shoots through the roof.

"Always keep your faith up."–Luzemily Prosper (11 years old)

- **Look 10 years younger**
  The way that this program turns back the clocks of time, as for your appearance, will be nothing short of amazing.

- **Feel 10 times stronger**
  Women will protect themselves from osteoporosis because, once you begin progressive weight resistance gradually and systematically, your bones become more dense and thus stronger and more resistant.

- **Live 10 years longer**
  Barring your getting hit by a truck or falling out of a window, you can expect to add years onto your otherwise natural life span.

You can change your appearance and physical condition in just 30 – 45 minutes each day. This is the last get-in-shape, lose-weight book you will ever need – *ever!*

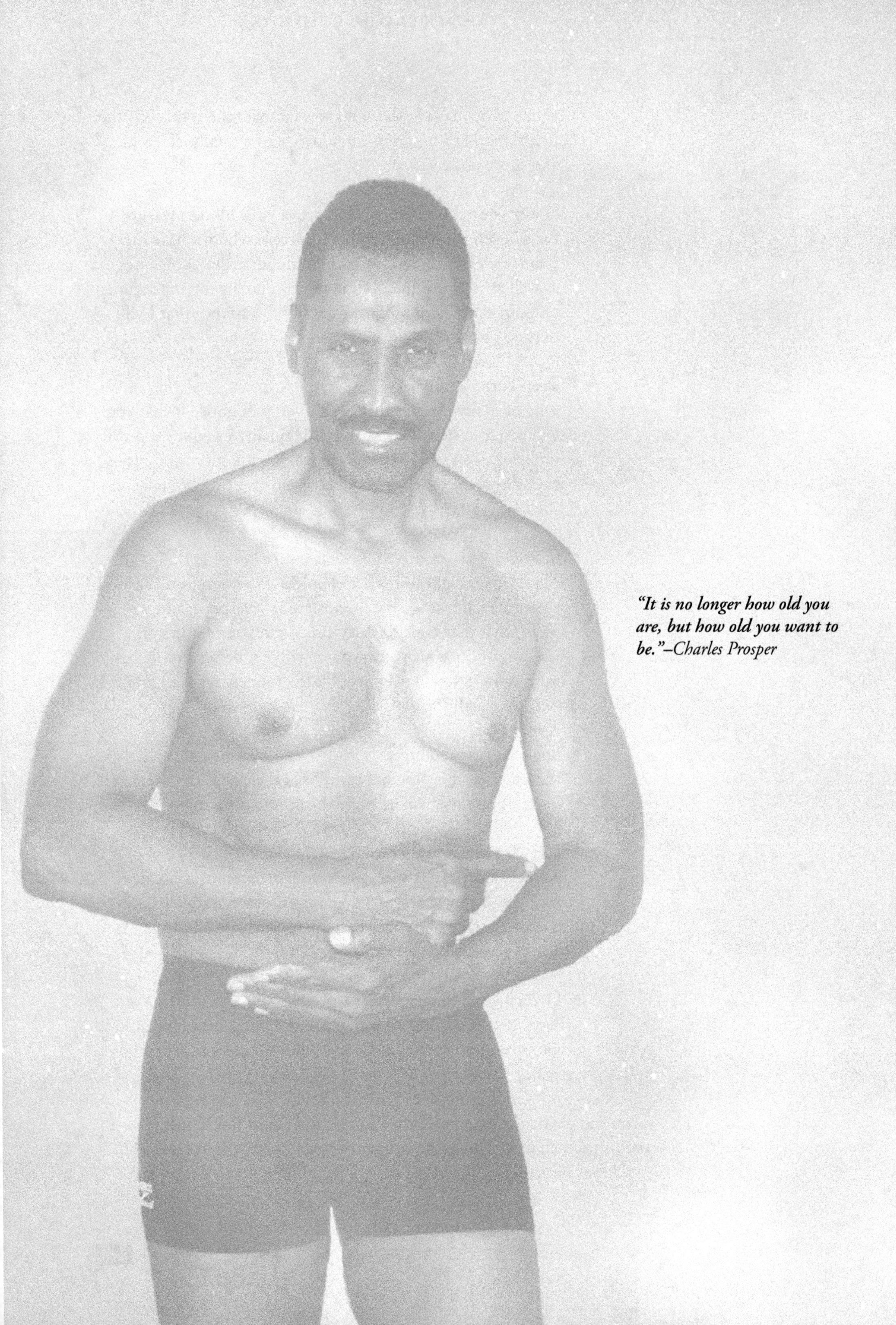

"It is no longer how old you are, but how old you want to be."–Charles Prosper

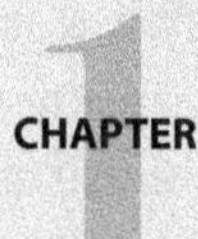
CHAPTER 1

My Story: From Fat To Fit

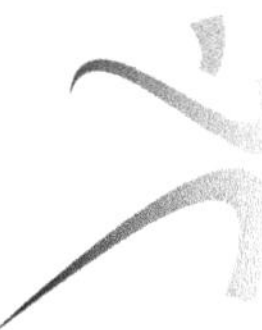

"Think you can, think you can't; either way, you'll be right."–Henry Ford

Who am I? Well, first of all, I am not a Mr. Universe. I am not a former Mr. America. I am only Mr. Prosper – a success story, who at age 50 realized that, body-wise, things were getting worse, and not any better. I was 35 lbs. over-weight, tired, unenergetic and rapidly going down hill. I had not done any serious physical exercise since I was around my mid-thirties. So, starting my journey of physical transformation after the mid-century mark, I am definitely a guy you can identify with, that is, if I can do it, you can do it also.

I had tried a few fad diets here and there, and as to be expected, all of them failed. The weight went off quickly, in fact *too* quickly, and as soon as I stopped, guess what? – yes, you got it, *fats-ville* once more.

So, I began to think "There's *got* to be a better way!" So, I asked myself who were the guys who had the most muscular bodies and maintained the least amount of body fat? People who practice body building! Of course. This was the correct route for me to go. Now, I wasn't interested in becoming a professional body-builder, but I did want to discover some of the secrets that they know which the average person doesn't. So, I did my research. Joined a gym and began to pay the monthly fees. But I noticed something: I was paying every month, but I wasn't going every day. In fact, I wasn't going but maybe once or twice a week. Then it reduced to one a week, then once every two weeks. Once a month. Soon I was paying the monthly gym fees, automatically taken out of my checking account, all the while trying to convince myself that I was going to go back – next month. After over twelve months of kidding myself, I decided to quit my gym membership and just buy a home gym which consisted of a bench, barbells and dumbbells. Now, I didn't have to pay a fee every month, and I didn't have to get up, go out and drive to an outside gym. Only, one problem, I put this gym set under my bed and in the closet where it sat for over one year. I'm not kidding you!

My Turning Point - That Which Got Me Serious

Well, obviously something happened to make me change these slothful ways, or I wouldn't be sitting here writing this book. Something did happen. My turning point happened when one day my then 7 year-old daughter said: "Daddy, I'll race you to the car." We both fired off for barely what was less 40 or 50 feet to see who'd reach the car door first, but only after a few seconds into the run, I was panting, gasping, huffing and puffing like the big, bad wolf with a case of asthma. *That* did it for me! I said to myself, with a true and sudden resolve, that there was *no* way that I would allow myself to deteriorate physically any further. I thought about my daughter. I had her when I was 50 years old. What this suddenly meant to me was that I needed to do my part, whatever it took, to stay healthy and live longer to be there for her as long as God's grace would let me. This meant that I had to cut the B.S. and get serious about taking care of my body and my health. It was at that moment and on that day that I said to myself, "Never again would I just sit back and allow myself to disappear ahead of time for the sake of my baby girl." Now was the time. On that same night, I pulled out those weights from under the bed. The next day, I had a friend to assemble my workout bench, and I was ready to go.

Finding The Right Time for Me To Exercise

"Genius is an infinite capacity for taking pains."–Jane Ellis Hopkins

Now, I started my exercise routine in earnest. I had my weights in the corner of the living room, but this was not convenient as it made our living space a little too crowded. The answer. I then decided to take all of my weights out into the back to our garden. This idea worked out just fine, and to my surprise, I found that weights and the basic workout equipment such as the benches and the power stands for squats hold up quite well in outside weather. Even after the rain, weights rust very little and if at all it is just a little superficial rust which can be wiped away with products like Rustoleum.

Things were going fine until I realized that exercising at 5:00 p.m. after a work day was beginning to get more and more difficult. My daughter needed help with her homework. I had to take her to volleyball practice after school, and with puppy-dog eyes she begged me to stay and watch her practice. In the afternoons, I also had to prepare dinner and get things ready for the next day. E-mail customer requests was also in no short supply in the late afternoons and evenings. What's a determined health enthusiast to do?

I had to find the *one* time of the day when I know that there would be no interruptions. Hence, for the last four years, my workout time is at 4:30 a.m. in the morning. I'm not kidding you! Now, don't get me wrong, it was not easy. I *hated* getting up at that time of morning in the first 3 weeks, but I began to think of the paraplegic paralysed from the neck down who would *gladly* love to trade places with me to have the opportunity to get up at all. You see, I am not saying that you have to get up in the predawn like me to exercise, but what I am saying is that it is not a burden to find time to exercise, it is a privileged blessing to be able to do so. The point is, whatever the time you select, it is the time that you must commit to. No excuses. Either you want better health, a longer life and a happier future, or you don't.

My Mentor - Melvin Powers

Everyone can look back to someone who played a pivotal part in sky-rocketing them to the success of their goal achievement. These people are called mentors. In my case, my mentor was Melvin Powers, better known as "The Mail Order Millionaire". Melvin is publisher of the Wilshire Book Company in Chatsworth, California. Melvin is the person who is responsible for motivating me to start my own publishing company, but beyond that, Melvin is now in his eighties, works out regularly with weights, and has the fitness of a forty-year old. I once saw him lift up his T-shirt, and all I saw was nothing but an incredible six-pack. Because of my age-bracket and being of the baby-boomer generation, *I love to encourage the middle-age man or woman*, that is, those over 40, 50 and 60. However, these health principles are not just for those of 50 and older. These health principles are for *anyone*, at any age, male or female, who is committed to becoming fabulously fit.

"Mediocrity knows nothing higher than itself, but talent instantly recognizes genius." – *Arthur Conan Doyle*

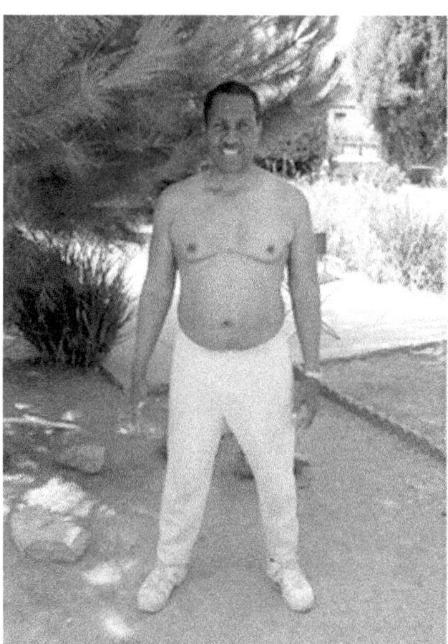

Me Before

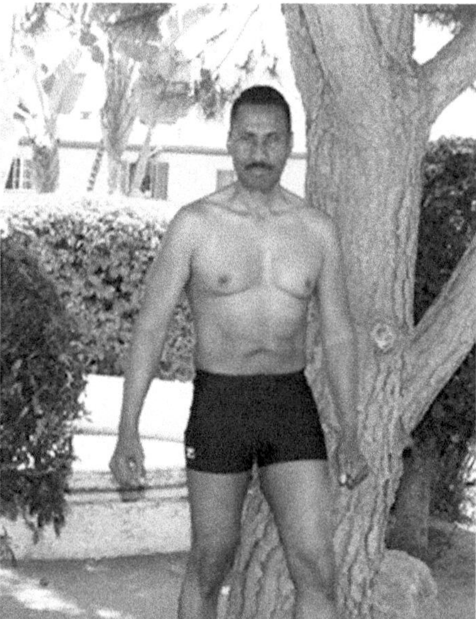

Me Today

So, no matter what your age or how you want to start, be it from home or a professional gym, I will show you how to reach your goal of total body fitness, such that if you are fifty, you will become fabulous, and if you are sixty, I will show you how to make sixty look *sexy*.

Remember, *it is no longer how old you are, but how old you want to be.*

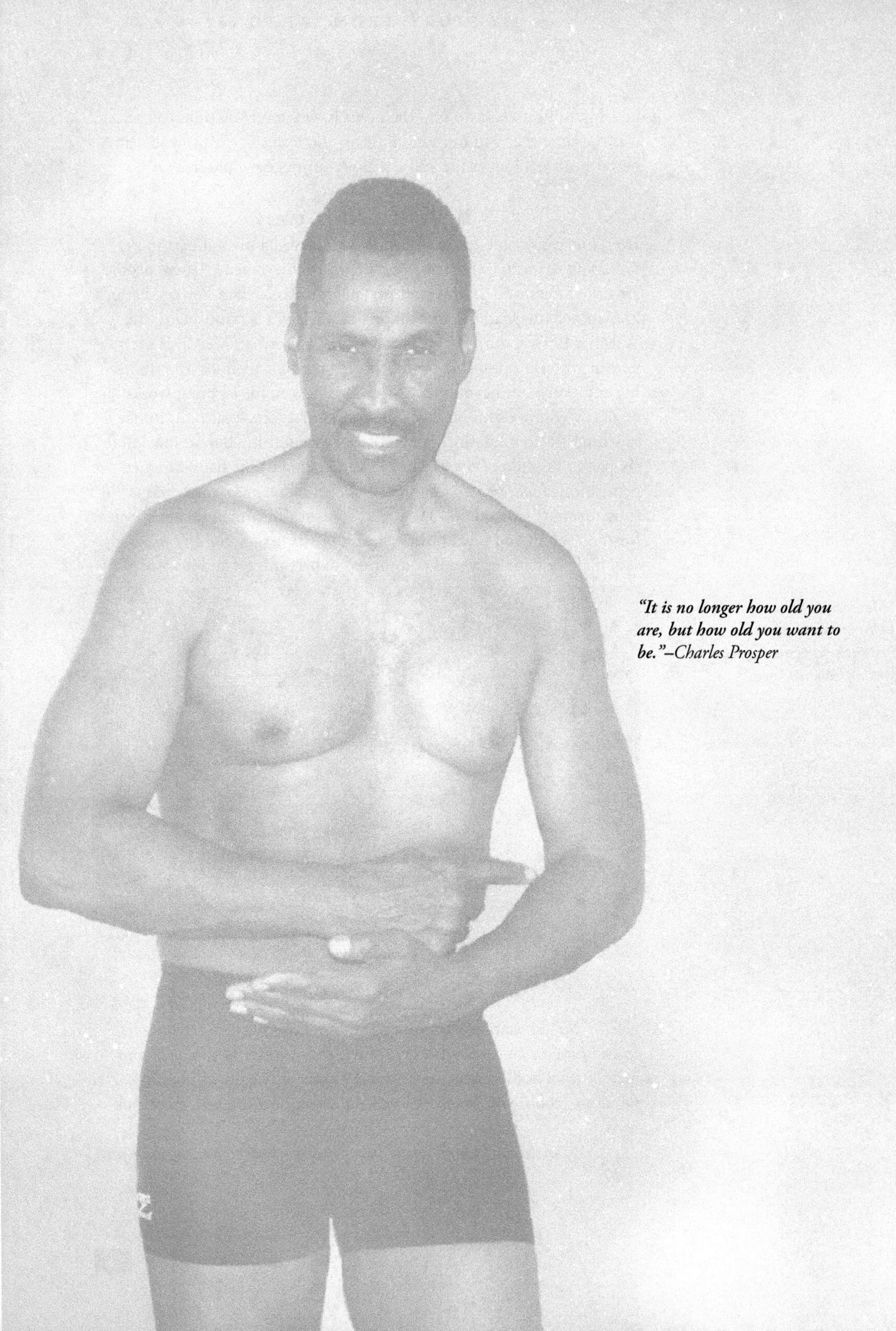

"It is no longer how old you are, but how old you want to be."–Charles Prosper

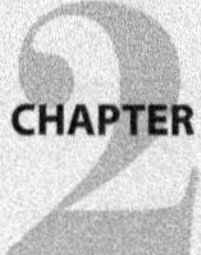

CHAPTER 2

Desire – It All Starts With Wanting To Change

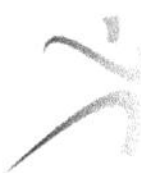

I want to make something perfectly clear. I am not on a crusade to make all fat people thin and all unhealthy people healthy. I can love anyone just as they have decided to be. They still have a soul, and if you want to talk about what really matters, that would be it. But even with that said, I do feel that I have a mission in the sense that I have something to give in the way of example, knowledge and the ability to convey complex concepts in a very simple format enough for you to see and believe that not only you can do, but to get you motivated and fired up to *continue* to do it. But it must start with something deep within you. That something deep within you is a decision made that is fueled by a strong desire to do something to become better than you are now.

"Be like a postage stamp– stick to one thing until you get there."–Josh Billings

It All Starts With Desire

How much do you want to change? Really. How much do you *really* want it? The intensity of your desire for change will determine your ability to persist in the face of delays, distractions and setbacks. As you have probably already surmised, my mantra and clarion call is *"It is no longer how old you are but how old you want to be."* This is more than a cute and catchy statement. It is truth. With the secrets and system that I will offer for you here, you will find that this statement is absolute truth if you will only follow through for only 12 weeks and see what happens.

Start By Taking a "Before" Photo

Nothing will motivate you to stay on track more than seeing proof in the form of visible change. You need to see from where you are beginning. So the first and most important thing that I can strongly recommend for you to do is to take a "before" photo the minute that you have truly decided to start. I suggest that you have someone take a color photo of you in your swimming attire, be it your swimming trunks if you are a guy or a bathing suit if you're a lady. It doesn't matter at all if fat is falling out all over the place. That's the fun of taking the "before" photo – to later see how far you have progressed. When you take your photos, you should take a front pose with your hands simply hanging at your sides. Take also a side angle photo, and a rear shot. It's okay if you look a little sad or shy in the photo as that will change when your "after" photo shows a beaming smile of success painted all over your face.

Measure Your Waistline Now – And Keep A Pair of The Pants You Wear

Though I am not a fanatic of excessive body parts measurements, because I feel that if you look good in the mirror and fit well in your clothes, it doesn't really matter what your measurements are. But I do believe that two measurements will be found to be both interesting and encouraging. Measure your waistline and weigh yourself. Now with a caveat, I ask you to weigh yourself in the beginning to have a point of reference, but changes in body weight in and of itself is not the best criteria to see how you have progressed. What I mean is this. Muscle weighs more than fat. It is quite possible to lose 10 lbs of body fat and gain 15 lbs of muscle at the same time. Sure you will, on the basis of just the scale, be 5 lbs heavier, but because you have shed ugly fat and have added more shapely muscle, you will look leaner and trimmer and totally, totally *awesome!* Mirrors don't lie. If you like what you see in the mirror, you are home free. However, even with that caveat, it will be very interesting to see how many inches you lose off of your waistline as well as see how your weight changes at the end of the 12 weeks. And as a success trophy or pirates booty, keep a pair of your pants that you use today to remember all of the person that used to go in there.

"Nothing great was ever achieved without enthusiam."–Ralph Waldo Emerson

Take Progress Photos of Yourself Every Two Weeks

Change will happen so rapidly that you will need to record your progress as quick as possible. Not only do I suggest that you take photos of yourself before you begin training, I recommend that you also take progress photos of yourself *every two weeks*. At the end of your 12 weeks, you will be an inspiration for others who will surely seek out your help as well.

In The Beginning, Sometimes You Just Won't Feel Like Exercising

It is difficult to form new habits when they go contrary to others that have been deeply ingrained and are diametrically opposite. The beginning of any new discipline involves suffering. I can't put it any other way. You must be willing to push yourself through the discomfort of the natural resistance to form and establish a new habit that involves work. The good news is that it only takes about 3 weeks of discipline before the habit phase sets in and what was initially a "new forced discipline" now becomes a pleasurable habit that is then so much a part of your life that you now *look forward* to doing it, and your body and mind wants more of it. But what are some tips to overcome the pain of inertia?

Just Dressing To Workout Will Help Put You In The Mood

I have found that another routine, innocuous in nature, that is tied to your doing your daily exercises will trigger a readiness and mood swing in favor of just doing it. Let me explain. Let us say that it is your third or fourth day of your routine, and you already are beginning to try to talk yourself out of working out today for postponing it until tomorrow. (Yeah *right!*)

Anyway, here is a little secret tip. Don't try to tell yourself that you are going to do a workout, just tell yourself and give yourself the permission to *just dress to go workout* – that's all. So, you dress with your sweats, tennis shoes and workout gloves. No problem. *Now*, that you have managed to put on your workout clothes, just convince yourself and give yourself the permission to walk out onto the workout floor. (If it is a home gym, go to your workout area; if it is a membership gym, get in the car, drive to the gym and walk on the floor.) So far, so good? Now just touch the weights. Are you okay? Good. Now, pick up a weight and see if you can do just one set of 10 repetitions of any one of your programmed exercises. Did one set? Okay, do just a second set. Wow! Congratulations. You did two sets! Oh, what the heck! Just do a third set. I can almost promise you that, at this stage, you will have shaken off all of the procrastination cobwebs, and you will find yourself in the midst of a productive and fruitful workout.

"Well begun is half done."– *Aristotle*

Select A Best Time Of Day To Exercise – And Stick To It

There is nothing that slows down your acclimation to your new routine more than not selecting and sticking to a best time of day to exercise, at least in the first 4 weeks. Your entirely mental and physical biorhythms begin to adjust and to prepare itself for that certain time of day that you have selected. What I am trying to say is that, if you just select and stick to a certain time to workout, at that particular chosen time, after about a few weeks, you will just *feel like exercising* – effortlessly. Our entire physiological organism is ruled by cycles and biorhythms. The body is always willing and ready to adjust if you will only give it a reliable pattern or cycle to follow.

Just Don't Skip

If I can give you any rule to follow when it comes to starting your discipline, establishing your new healthy success habits and that would be simply this. Just don't skip! Don't skip, if at all possible, any of your workouts. Remember, this is not something you are doing to get something and stop. You are forming a new life style. Exercise is now becoming part of your regular daily life style. Just as you plan to eat everyday of your life, or sleep every day of your life or bathe every day of your life, you will now have a new category, exercise everyday of your life. If you can only do half of your workout routine, then for God's sake, only do half. Just don't skip.

The Young And Muscular Sexagenarian On Venice Beach

I am sure that most of you have heard of Venice Beach, California. This is the famed "Muscle Beach" where the footsteps of some of the most recognized professional body builders have ever walked its sands. Though nowadays Venice Beach is not as populated with the famous body builders of the past, you do get to see a lot of incredibly muscular and fit individuals work out in the nearby Gold's Gym. I was completely blown away by a man in his sixties with a muscularity and "six pack" of abs that was tantamount to a muscular gymnast in his twenties. I was speechless. I asked him his "secret". Instead of telling me of some spectacular exercise routine or some nutritional supplements that only a select few knew about, he gave me his secret in one word. He said: "Consistency." He said: "No matter what routine you select, be consist about it." This lesson has always stuck with me.

Later I heard someone say this quote, a motivational speaker whom I cannot recall at this time, but the quote is significant to what I am saying here. He said: *"Ordinary things consistently done produce extraordinary results."*

***"See things as you would have them instead of as they are."**–Robert Collier*

Don't Tell Anyone What You Are Doing

Would you like a fun tip to keep you motivated and be an inspiration to others? In the beginning, don't talk about what you are going to do. Why? For two good reasons:

1) It weakens your resolve.

2) You expose yourself to the negativity of others.

Talking about an important project before you have embarked upon it weakens your resolve because you are unwittingly looking for outside external validation that you are doing the right thing. Why does anybody tell someone about an important and difficult project that they are about to undertake? For "other person validation". You want to hear: "Wow! That's great. Congratulations!" This is what you would like to hear, but that is not always what you get. And even if 20 people said it was a good idea, at this stage, you would have become addicted to hearing the approval of others because there is no concept of "enoughness" when it comes to seeking others' approval. Just by law of probability, sooner or later you will come across that 21st or 22nd person who will say: "You don't need to do all of that. It's a waste of time and money. Just watch what you eat, and you will be fine." Now, the minute you get a negative comment, you try to defend your reasons, and let me tell you a secret, whenever you try to defend your beliefs out of fear, you weaken your resolve even more.

When you talk about your good plans, you expose yourself to the negativity of others. And if you believe that there are no negative (overweight themselves) people who would just love to see you fail, you are in for a very rude awakening. Just don't talk about it to anyone. Let your results speak for themselves.

"I think and think for months and years. Ninety-nine times the conclusion is false. The hundredth time I am right"–*Albert Einstein*

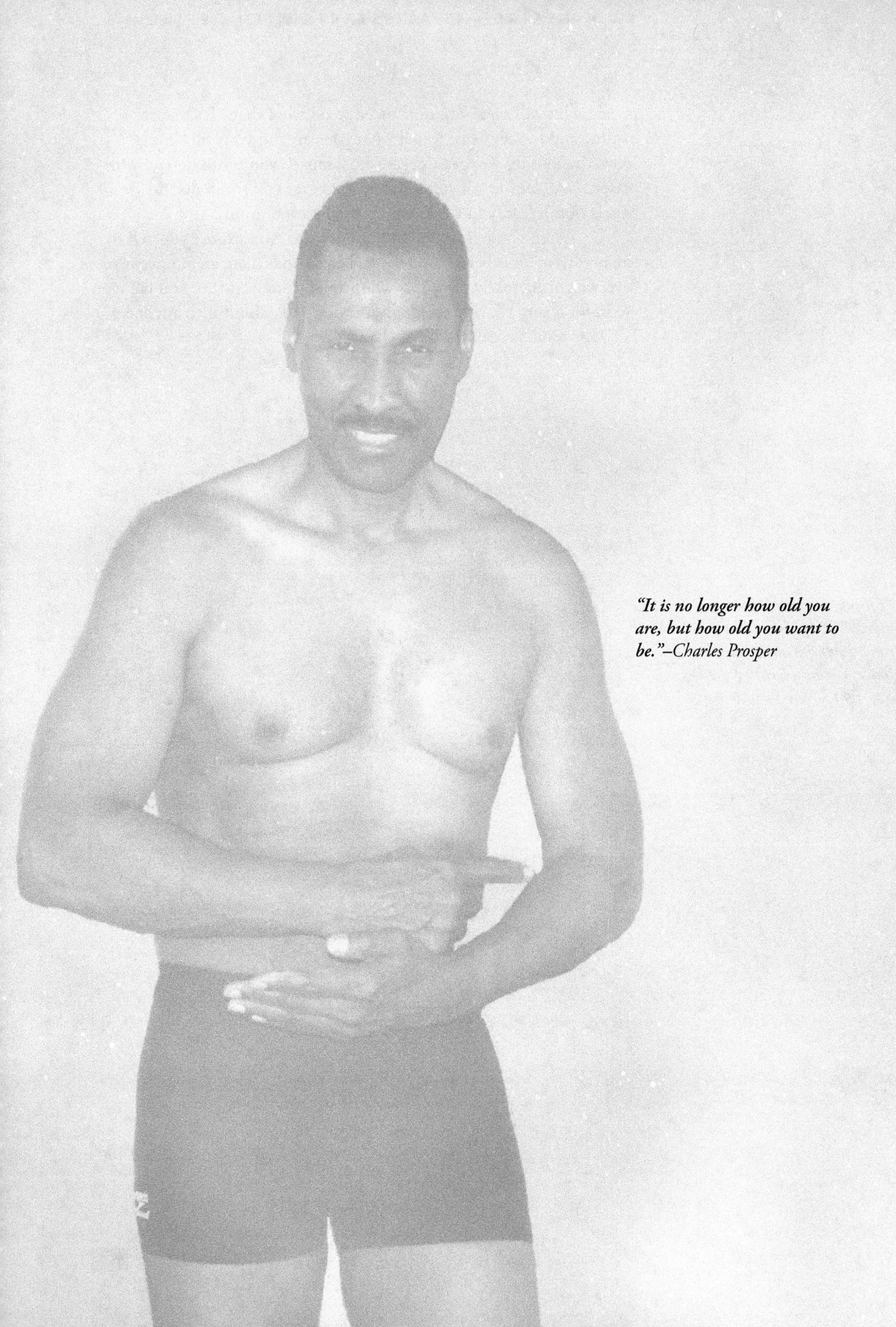

"It is no longer how old you are, but how old you want to be."–Charles Prosper

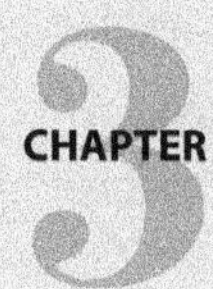

CHAPTER 3

The Prosper Fit Fast System

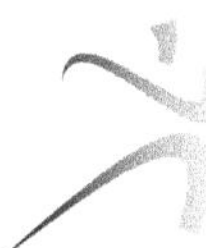

"Never stop. One always stops as soon as something is about to happen."–Peter Brook

Now I would like to formally introduce you to your key to get fit fast. I call this "The Prosper Fit Fast System". This system has five proven and easy components that makes it work all of the time and for anyone when it is done consistently – no matter what your age is or what shape you are in.

The Prosper Fit Fast System

Briefly, these are the 5 key elements of this 12-week and for life program:

- Progressive Weight Resistance
- Clean, Healthy Eating (No Dieting)
- Eat 5 Small But Nutritious Meals A Day
- "Cheat-Eat" One Day A Week
- Aerobics (20 minutes) Every 3rd Day

Progressive Weight Resistance

Though diet is one of the major cornerstones of your success as well as exercise. The *type* of exercise that you select is also crucially important. I am going to speak in absolutes now at the risk of rubbing some people the wrong way, but that's okay. I can handle it. The absolute best way to strengthen your body, shape your muscles, sculpt your figure, accelerate your fat-burning metabolism, strengthen your heart and virtually turn back the clocks of time to regain a youth and energy that you thought you had lost forever is, without doubt, hands down, *progressive weight resistance.*

The usual components of progressive weight resistance are barbells and dumbbells as well as a variety of fancy machines and equipment. But here, I would like to keep it simple. You will notice that the types of progressive weight resistance exercises that I feature here in this book basically consists of barbells, dumbbells and a workout bench.

If you are really serious, these basic pieces of equipment are all you really need. You do not need the latest fad piece of miracle-working exercise equipment that you just saw on a TV informercial "*...for only six easy payments of $150.00".* I believe in the KISS Principle. (Keep It Simple Student.)

You can easily create your own home gym with less that $250 to start, or you can enroll in your neighborhood membership gym.

Clean Healthy Eating (No Diets)

My mother and father taught me that an educated person never has the need to use four letter words or vulgarity. I hope that they forgive me now for I am about to use a "four-letter word" – diet. Diets are profane. Diets don't help. Diets don't work.

First of all, let us understand the true meaning of diet as most people use it. "I need to lose 30 lbs. I can't squeeze into these jeans anymore. I need to go on a diet." What is this person really saying? He or she is saying that they want to radically and *temporarily* change their eating habits for the purpose of losing 30 lbs. But tacitly within this same statement is the unconscious acceptance, that once the 30 lbs. are lost, one will resume his or her "normal" eating patterns again. Thus the body realizes that the weird "food famine" is over and will happily replace the weight that was removed plus a little more to be prepared for the next "famine".

"Life is too short to read bad books."–Charles Prosper

When you reduce calories and fat *without* exercise, the "body consciousness" interprets this as some sort of sudden starvation and attempts to end its existence. (These are the body's "thoughts", mind you.) So, what does the body do when you put it on a diet? It *slows* the metabolism down conserving all the fat "energy reserves" as it can during this "famine". Though you will lose weight quickly on many radical diets, at the same time, you are training your metabolism to hold on to as many fat cells as possible in the process. Once you have lost those 30 lbs. or so in this radical manner, when you resume normal eating, the tendency now is to gain weight even faster than when you started your diet. Why? Now your body, through the time you were on the diet, has transformed itself into a fat-storing machine. This is why most people, after a diet is over, gain it all back rather quickly with a little extra to boot.

Clean, healthy eating has nothing to do with dieting. Clean, healthy eating is not designed to be extreme nor as a *temporary* regime. Clean, healthy eating is just a new way of life where you eat good, nutritious, delicious and satisfying meals with no feeling of suffering nor sacrifice. You will be able to eat lean and clean for life – and love it. With *The Prosper Fit Fast System*, we don't call eating "dieting" – *not ever* – you have only changed the *way* and *what* you eat.

Eat 5 Small Meals A Day

You are now in for a surprise and for a treat. To lose your maximum amount of body fat in the fastest and safest way, as well as developing shapely and sexy looking muscles, I will show you how to eat not less but *more* meals every day – and you will never feel hungry nor unsatisfied.

The problem with the way the most of us in modern day society have learned to eat is via the 3 square meals a day paradigm. The problem with this form of eating is that breakfast is either skipped, overdone or eaten improperly. Lunch is usually too heavy with an over emphasis on sandwiches, and dinner can be a virtual pig-out, especially when a rich high-calorie dessert is indulged in to finish it off.

Let's look at what can happen just at breakfast. The worst that can happen is if you skip it. You are hungry from not having eaten for 6 to 8 hours after awakening. Your metabolism is also high and ready to digest food. But what happens, you skip it, thus creating even more hunger with the great chance of over-eating at lunch-time. You can also do your body great damage by eating a crappy breakfast. An example? How about a chocolate eclair or doughnut and coffee? Do you have any idea what this "sugar dump" on an empty stomach will do to your body in the morning? For one it will spike (raise) your blood insulin causing your body to go into a mild insulin shock which will trigger your fat storage mechanism. You will sometimes feel nervous and jittery the entire morning long. (This is how to make your kid hyper before school - just give her a couple of doughnuts and juice, and I promise you, her teacher will be calling you to get her off of the ceiling at school.)

"We cannot direct the wind, but we can adjust the sails."–Anonymous

And if excess sugar weren't enough in the morning to start your day wrong, how about a few strips of bacon with those hash browns and eggs over easy? Having clogged arteries, high blood pressure and stroke is a very heavy price to enjoy you daily grease. In the end, the pig will get his sweet revenge.

Now if you skip breakfast and lunch and try to "make it up" at dinner time, you might as well start wearing elastic waist ban pants to work because sooner or later, if you wear regular pants with a belt, people at work will shout one day : *"Everybody duck! It's going to blow!"*

So, what is the secret to avoid this food travesty? Simple. Eat every 3 hours. That is, eat 5 small but nutritious meals roughly every three hours. And let me define meal for you. Anything that you put in your mouth is called a *meal.* Just as a *bowl of grits, 4 scrambled egg whites, and a half an apple* is a meal for breakfast, so is considered a meal for mid-morning *non-fat cottage cheese, blueberries and a handful of almonds* as well. If you eat a mid-afternoon *protein power bar and two cups of water*, this too is called a *meal.*

The schedule of your five meals a day might look like this:

- **Breakfast** – 7:00 a.m.
- **Mid-Morning Meal** – 10:00 a.m.
- **Lunch** – 12:00 p.m.
- **Mid-Afternoon Meal** – 3:00 p.m.
- **Dinner** – 6:00 p.m.

What you will notice, will be the change of how you organize and plan your meals. One of the keys to making the system of eating 5 small meals work is that you will have to learn to plan your meals ahead of time, just like you will learn to plan your exercise workout routines, by say, getting your meals ready the night before. You will soon be known as the person with the biggest lunch box at your work place. You will need something to carry at least three meals: your mid-morning meal, your lunch and your mid-afternoon meal. Your co-workers will begin to admire you and start proclaiming that they too need to start bringing their lunch to work - of course which they rarely ever do.

"There is no such thing as a problem without a gift...you seek problems because you need their gifts."–Richard Bach

There are other benefits of taking the trouble to plan, prepare and carry your meals around ready with you. You will save money by not having to pay for expensive cafeteria and heart-clogging fast food at the corner burger place.

It will take a few weeks to get used to eating like this, but after it becomes a habit, you will never want to go back to your old fast food eating ways.

"Cheat-Eat" One Day A Week

"Cheat-eat" one day a week? What on God's earth could I be talking about here? You will now be rewarded for your self-discipline and dedication on your clean eating path. Pick one day of the week. If you like Sundays, on that day, eat whatever you want for any one meal of that day that you wish. If you want to have a lunch with a hamburger and fries – go for it! Are you looking at that chocolate fudge cake with vanilla ice cream on top in the dessert menu? Why resist? Enjoy every chocolate crumb of that cake. Something very interesting happens once you are strict and disciplined all week long and you allow yourself a "cheat-day" with a "cheat-meal". You body is becoming metabolically efficient for fat burning. You have trained it well. When you take one day and one meal and "cheat", that is, eat whatever you want, your body takes this as a mistake or fluke in your eating habits. So, what does the body do? It will actually *turn up* the metabolic fat-burning process, interpreting these high-caloric foods as a weekly mistake. As long as you resume your regular regime of lean, clean eating from Monday through Saturday, that Sunday "cheat meal" will not affect you at all. Some people actually *lose* weight after a "cheat meal" when they resume their exercises the next day! One last thing – eat *first* your portion of protein.

Aerobics (20 Minutes) Every 3rd Day

When I get to the chapter on weight training exercises, I will explain to you in detail the system of alternating progressive weight training with aerobics or cardio as it is sometimes known. But briefly, this is a possible example of your schedule of exercise:

Monday: (A Routine) – Chest, Shoulders, Triceps

Tuesday: (B Routine) – Back, Biceps, Forearms

• *Wednesday: (X Routine) – 20 minutes of cardio*

Thursday: (C Routine) – Legs, Abdominals

Friday: (A Routine) – Chest, Shoulders, Triceps

• *Saturday: (X Routine) – 20 minutes of cardio*

Sunday: (B Routine) – Back, Biceps, Forearms

Monday: (C Routine) – Legs, Abdominals

• *Tuesday: (X Routine) – 20 minutes of cardio*

Wednesday: (A Routine) – Chest, Shoulders, Triceps

Thursday: (B Routine) – Back, Biceps, Forearms

• *Friday: (X Routine) – 20 minutes of cardio*

"Your success is only as good as the excuses you refuse to live by."–Charles Prosper

Can you see the pattern here? Every *third* day, you do 20 intense minutes of aerobics or cardio exercises.

How To Do Aerobics for Maximum Fat-Burning

Let me show you how to get maximum fat-burning effect from your 20-minutes of aerobic activity on the third day following the two consecutive days of weight training.

The types of aerobic activity are varied. You can do stationary bicycling, treadmill walking, or my favorite, jogging outside with all of nature surrounding me.

There are several keys to successful aerobic exercise for maximum fat-burning.

The Keys To Effective Fat-Burning Aerobics:

1. **Do** your cardio exercise over 20 minutes but less than 45 minutes.

2. **Run**, walk, or bicycle on an *empty* stomach, preferably upon awakening in the morning which is when you will trigger the *maximum* fat-burning effect. Since you haven't eaten for 6 or 8 hours, your body is hungry and your metabolism begins to trigger and readies to burn fat. When you go, for example, outside and begin to jog, for the first 20 minutes, your body will quickly burn up your blood glucose and glycogen for energy. What is glucose? Glucose is a type of sugar found in the blood. The blood carries glucose to every cell in the body, for use as energy. What is glycogen? Glycogen is a main source of stored energy in the body. Glycogen is stored primarily in liver and muscle cells. This glucose and glycogen store usually depletes after the 20-minute mark. Go just 5 more minutes, and your body begins to voraciously burn body fat, which is what you want. Your stored body fat will begin to emulsify and just melt off your body. And here's the beautiful thing of it all. This accelerated, fat-burning metabolic activity continues for hours *after* you have finished exercising. And how can you know this for certain? Well, I will let you in on a little secret. You will find yourself with frequent and very strong urges to urinate for the first few hours after exercising. You see, your body is eliminating the emulsified fat cells through your urine. So, every time you have the strong urge to urinate, you are urinating fat cells. Melted fat cells are *also* eliminated every time you have a bowel movement as well. If you are eating properly with the right amount of fiber, your bowel movements will increase also.

"All you need is a plan, a road map and the courage to press on to your destination."–Earl Nightingale

3. **Drink** a cup of coffee (sweetened with Splenda if you like) or a cup of hot green tea just before you jog, on an empty stomach, of course. Let me interject here that when I say "on an empty stomach", I would like to clarify it with saying that "on an empty stomach" includes after you have drunk two cups of fresh water upon awakening *before* you drink your cup of coffee or your cup of green tea. (Coffee has a slight diuretic effect which means that because of the caffeine content, it causes the body to lose water. You don't want to dehydrate.) The caffeine in coffee has been shown to boost the metabolism when taken moderately, that is to speed up the fat-burning mechanism. Green tea also burns fat and boosts the metabolism, and unlike coffee, it doesn't leave your stomach with occasional acidity.

4. **Super-fat burning** secret! Take 2 tablespoons of liquid L-Carnitine which you can find at any nutrition or health store. L-Carnitine is an amino-acid based (amino-acids are the basic stuff of proteins), safe, and fast-acting fat-burning food supplement. To understand how L-Carnitine works, we have to go to cellular level and understand a part of the cell that is called the mitochondria. What the mitochondria is and does is that it is in essence the fat-burning furnace of the cells. When you take L-Carinitine, what it does, in essence is *push* the fat cells surrounding the muscle tissue *into* the area of the mitochondria. So, now your muscles are burning *fat* stored as energy! This is *so* cool! After waking up in the morning on your cardio day, start by drinking your two cups of fresh water, followed by your cup of coffee or green tea – and *then* take two tablespoons of liquid L-Carnitine. You are now revved up and ready as one mean, lean, fat-burning machine.

"Your life is only as good as the people you serve."–*Charles Prosper*

5. **Super-energy** secret! Drink a small vial of liquid Chinese ginseng right after the L-Carnitine. Get ready for some incredible power and energy. You will feel like flying after a few days of ginseng as part of your morning ritual. (This is also taken – empty stomach – as a pre-aerobic supplement.) Ginseng helps the body hold oxygen better - thus more energy.

6. **Jog** steady. Then fast. Then steady. I am using jogging as my example here for the aerobic activity, but it could likewise be stationary bicycling, or walking the treadmill plank at the gym. What I am giving you here is the secret to use aerobic or cardio activity for *maximum* fat-burning. The key word is *intensity*. This is what turns up the fat-burning furnace of aerobic activity. This is how it should be done. Let's stick with jogging as our example. The first 5 minutes, you jog at a moderate but steady pace. Then – *burst* out fast and run as fast as you can (without falling) for another 2 to 5 minutes. You should now be breathing quite heavily. Resume your jog at a moderate pace once more until your breathing normalizes. As soon as you catch your breath – *burst* out again for another 2 to 5 minutes. Keep this pattern up for 20 minutes or more, and you will be burning body fat like there is no tomorrow. Now this intensity pattern, of moderate, followed by fast, followed by moderate, followed by fast is indeed the best and the fastest way to burn fat. This is not to say, however, that by jogging moderately to begin, on a regular basis of even for 10 or 15 minutes, will show you no results, for it will. This slow-fast, slow-fast is just a little more efficient. You will get to your goal much faster. Warning: Be careful not to go beyond 45 minutes when doing aerobics or cardio on an empty stomach. Why? Because beyond 45 minutes, your body shifts from burning fat to burning precious muscle tissue by using up the amino acids found in the protein of your muscle tissue that should only be used for muscle growth and body recuperation. This is the bottom line. The more muscle you grow, the more your body becomes a fat-burning machine. Muscle tissue tends to burn fat tissue even while it is at rest – hours after you have put your weights down. So, as a general rule, I would say that 30 minutes of slow-fast, slow-fast aerobic activity is perfect.

"We are Divine Personalities as part of God's divine dream of Himself."–Charles Prosper

Stages of Getting Used To Aerobic Activity If You Are Out of Shape

Stage 1 - Walk as fast as you can. 5 or 10 minutes is okay in the beginning.

Stage 2 - Walk as fast as you can. 20 to 25 minutes.

Stage 3 - Jog lightly. 10 to 15 minutes.

Stage 4 - Jog moderately - non-stop. 10 to 25 minutes.

Stage 5 - Jog quickly - non-stop. 25 minutes doing "slow-fast".

Take your time. Do your best. Doing your best is more important than being the best.

"A strong passion for any object will guarantee success, for the desire of the end will point to the means." *–William Hazlitt*

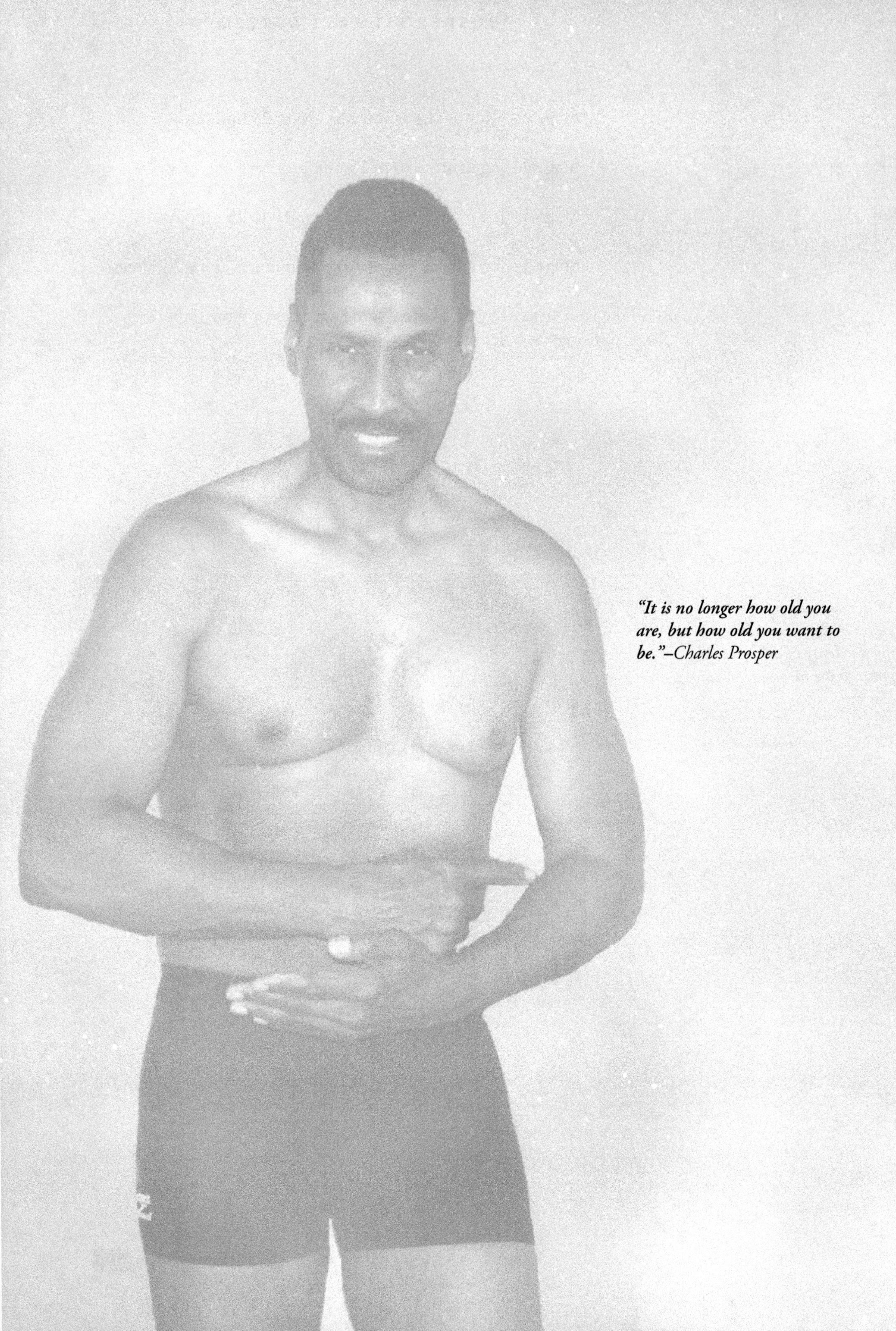

"It is no longer how old you are, but how old you want to be."–Charles Prosper

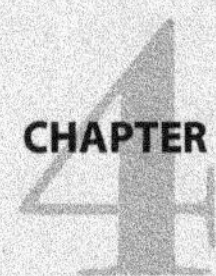

CHAPTER 4

Your Five Stages of Progress

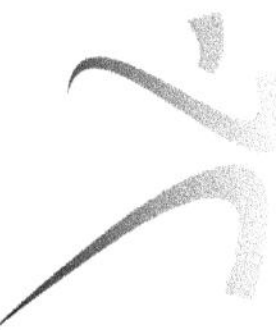

If you have never practiced progressive weight training, it would be nice to know what stages of progress you might expect. Though I am sure that someone with *way* too much information about the subject could complicate and make understanding these stages progress hard to understand, but I would like to keep things very simple and tell you that there are essentially 5 stages of progress that most people will go through.

"Everyone has a talent. What is rare is the ourage to follow that talent to the dark place where it leads."–Erica Jong

The Five Stages of Progress

Okay, let's take a look at what you might expect as you embark upon your maiden voyage from fat to fit.

Stage 1 – *Feeling Tired* You may feel a little tired during the first week of your exercise. This is normal if it happens to you. Your body is adapting to new and beneficial habits and to start almost anything new, there is an initial resistance. The remedy to this temporary condition is that you should get from 7 to 8 of hours sleep which will help your body to recuperate faster and build more muscle tissue.

Stage 2 – *Losing Stomach Bloat* During the second and third week, something very nice and surprising will happen. You will say goodbye to stomach bloat. All of the excess water that is retained, due to poor eating habits and lack of exercise will be flushed out, leaving your stomach flatter than it has been in years.

Stage 3 – *Very Frequent Urination* One of the sure signs that you are burning fat off of your body are the sudden and frequent urges to urinate after a full-body workout with weights. You see, fat cells are now being emulsified very rapidly by a newly charged up metabolism. Your fat is literally melting off of your body, and your body is eager to get rid of the wastes and toxins as soon as possible. Look at it on the bright side. Every time you rush to the bathroom, you are *urinating fat!*

Stage 4 – *Muscle Soreness* This may occur the day after you exercise or even on the *second* day after, that is, occasionally you may get sore two days after you have exercised with weights. Actually, soreness is a *good* thing. The reason for the soreness is that your muscles are in a repair state. Let me explain. When you do progressive weight resistance, you break down your old, weak and flabby muscle tissue which is literally washed away from the bloodstream. Now, on the next day, your body *replaces* the weak, broken down muscle and *adds* a little more muscle tissue, but the new muscle tissue is stronger and more athletic than the tissue you had just two days ago. So, look at it this way: rejoice when you wake up with a little muscle soreness the next day because this is the sure sign that your muscles are getting bigger and stronger. If you go to a professional bodybuilders gym, you will hear them bragging with glee at how sore they woke up from an evening of exercise the day before. When you are training intensely and heavy enough, you too will be blessed with soreness.

"There's a way to do it better...find it."–Thomas Edison

Stage 5 – *Have Energy All The Time* Somewhere around the 5th or 6th week (or sooner), you will find, that suddenly, you have energy all of the time. Also as your workouts become more intense, you will tend to do them faster thus your workout time will become shorter. You will be in and out of the gym in no time.

Don't Forget To Take Your "Before" Photo

I just can't say it enough. Take a before photo of yourself, and you will be *amazed* at how you'll look in 12 weeks. This is the last time to record how you look now. Changes will occur very rapidly. Put on your swim trunks or bathing suit, and take a photo from the front, side and rear. I would also suggest *at the very least* that you take a progress photo of yourself on the first of every month. By the third month, you are a totally new person. Keep on track, keep up your new fitness life style and check yourself out after a year. "Wow!" – you will *surely* say.

"Be like the eraser...forever forgiving."–Charles Prosper

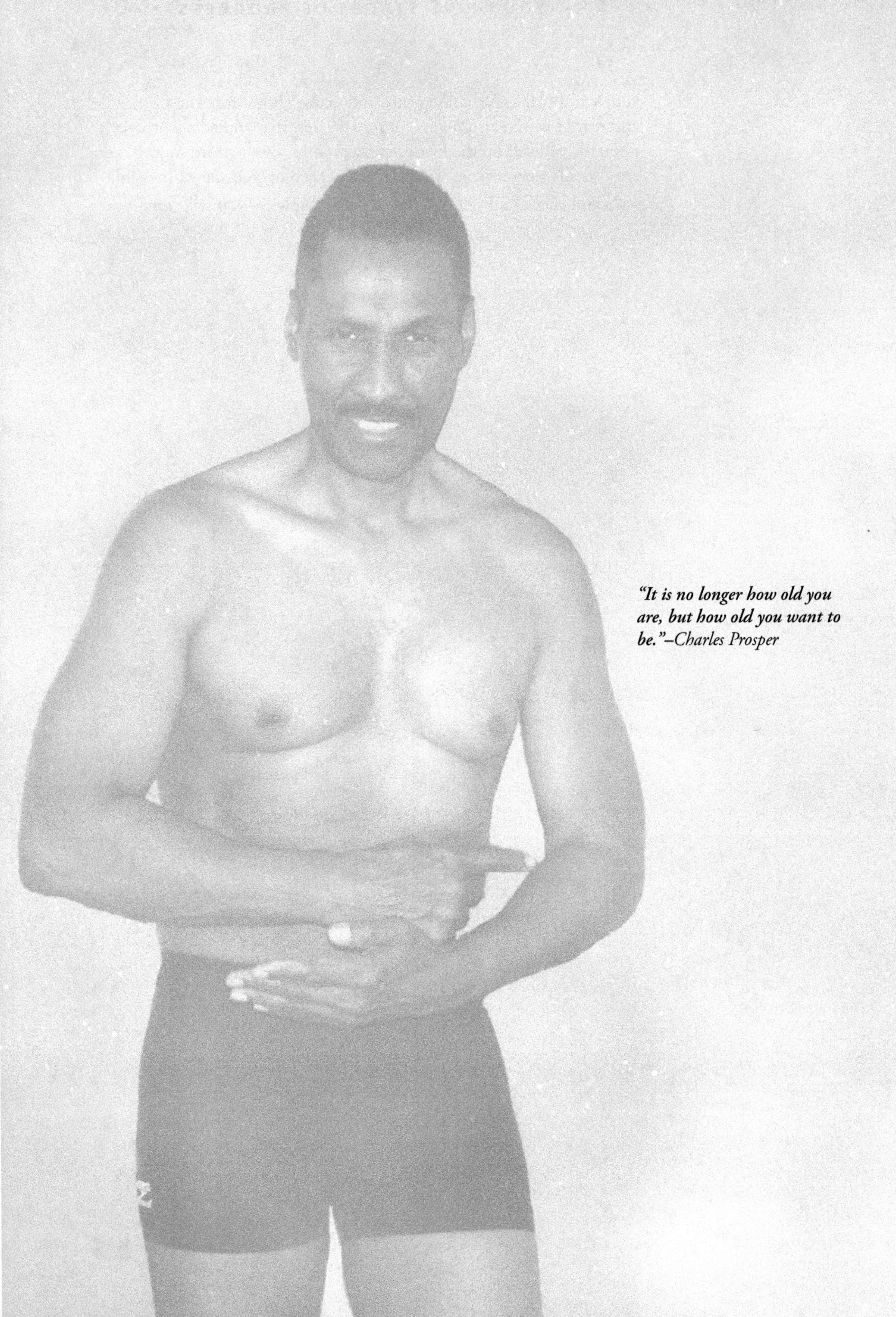

"It is no longer how old you are, but how old you want to be."–Charles Prosper

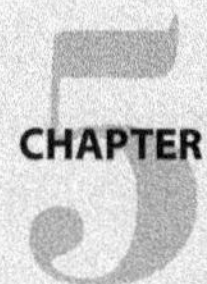

CHAPTER 5

The Best System For Permanent Weight Loss

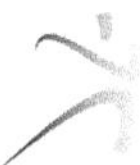

In this chapter, which deals with the best system for permanent weight loss, I am going to appear a bit biased. Biased is probably putting it mildly, but nevertheless, I am one who likes to shoot from the hip and tell it like it is. Before I tell you what I think is absolutely the one and only best system for permanent weight lost, I would first like to take a look at some of the popular and well known systems and paths to weight loss. However, before I go over each system one-by-one, I am itching right now to destroy a very popular myth concerning weight loss – spot reducing, that is doing an exercise that will reduce or take fat off certain areas of the body, like doing tons of sit ups with the hope and expectation that the fat will *specifically* melt off the stomach area.

"Why problems? If you are never given the opportunity, how can faith be developed?"–Charles Prosper

There Is No Exercise That Creates Spot Reducing

Let me say it one more time. There is no such thing as spot reducing. You cannot do sit ups and expect to have the fat drip off your stomach and no where else. Each person's body is uniquely and genetically pre-disposed to storing fat in a favorite spot. Maybe it's your thighs, or maybe it's your big butt. (Just teasing you.) When you exercise properly, you will lose weight all over your body, thus spot reducing will not be necessary, even though in some areas you *will* tend to lose faster than in others, but still the fat reduction is happening all over your body.

The Five Main Systems of Weight Loss and Physical Conditioning

- **Aerobics and Dieting**
- **Jogging and Dieting**
- **Dieting Only**
- **Diet Weight Loss Pills**
- **Progressive Weight Resistance, Cardio & Clean Eating**

Aerobics and Dieting

When I use the word aerobics here, I am including any sustained activity that will raise your heart rate and accelerate your breathing. Such exercises include as a partial list: stationary or outside bicycling, aerobic kickboxing, treadmill walking, stair climbing and more.

Jogging and Dieting

Well, yeah, I guess I could have included jogging along with the aerobics and dieting category, but to joggers, the really committed joggers, it is an exercise that is a class of its own. Still in all honesty, you could easily classify it along with the aerobics and dieting category.

Dieting Only

Oh, boy. In a bit, I will explain why this route spells trouble and guaranteed frustration. Millions of people everyday try this method, and to their surprise but not to mine, they always fail. In a moment, I will explain why diets are inherently set up for failure no matter who the "Dr." is that is espousing it.

"I start where the last man left off."–Thomas Edison

Dieting Weight-Loss Pills

I *still* find it hard to believe that there are still so many people who think that popping a pill will solve their woes. Pharmaceutical companies are always coming up with the "diet weight-loss pill d'jour", and later results almost always show that it was never what it was reported to be. Sure, weight loss does occur, but usually at the expense of your health and safety. Diet pills usually operate under the premise of artificial appetite suppression. The Wall Street Journal reported 18 million fen-phen prescriptions a month in 1996. The result. Heart-valve disease as a direct result of using fen-phen diet pills. All diet pills have negative side effects, some worse than others, some damaging to your health and others a threat to your life. Is it worth it if I can give you a safe and sure alternative?

Why Dieting Only Will Never Work

By definition, a diet is a *temporary* and radical food eating plan usually involving extreme calorie reduction over a short period of time. The operational word here is temporary. Diets are not meant to be stayed on forever. And this in and of itself is the problem. What happens when the diet is over and you have lost those 10, 20 or 30 lbs? You guessed it. You gain it all back and then a little more. Why? When you diet by just reducing calories in the absence of exercise, you unwittingly slow down your natural fat-burning metabolism because your body thinks that you are trying to starve it. So you indeed lose the weight this way, suffering through the hunger of it every minute.

But in the process, you have trained your metabolism *not* to burn fat very quickly, so it *slows* down – a whole lot. The minute you get off of your diet and resume normal eating, your body in an attempt to preserve itself for the next famine that you might put it through, now, *after* your diet, begins to store fat onto your body faster than you lost it. Thus in a short time, you gain it all back – and then some. Altogether now. Repeat after me – *"Diets don't work!"*

Why Just Aerobics or Jogging Are *Never* Enough

Look, let's get clear about something. You are not trying to lose fat *and* muscle tissue. However, this is exactly what you will do to yourself if you focus excessively on aerobics and/or jogging, jogging, jogging *ad infinitum, ad nauseam.* After doing an hour or more of aerobics or jogging, you will have used up your muscle glycogen for energy – then in a survival effort, your body will indiscriminately begin to burn up *both* fat *and* muscle tissue (bad news). You are in essence losing your natural fat-burning tissue, i.e., muscle – hence (and here comes the irony) – *your metabolism will now slow down.* Now pay close attention to this. When your metabolism slows down, you *gain* and retain fat – hence you attain the "Richard Simmons" type *chubby-aerobic-style* body. This is to say that with jogging or aerobics alone, if you are pear-shaped, you just become a slightly smaller shaped pear! So, then what is the answer to the healthy weight loss and body shaping conundrum?

"The mind is the limit. As long as the mind can envision the fact that you can do something, you can do it, as long as you really believe 100 percent." *–Arnold Schwarzenegger*

Progressive Weight Resistance, Cardio and Clean Eating

Forget everything else. This is your triad of physical fitness success. Weight training adds and *keeps* muscle while burning fat and giving your body a shaped and sexy look. Weight training shapes and sculpts your body by adding lean muscle tissue in just the right places giving you a more masculine or curvy feminine look.

Dr. Ronald Bahr of the National Institute of Occupational Health of Oslo, Norway, studied the effects of weight resistance exercise on the rate of fat metabolism after engaging in 30 minutes of intense weight resistance training. Dr. Bahr found that your body will burn fat for up to 12 hours *after you have finished exercise!* This means while you are sitting at the computer or just watching TV while sitting on the sofa – you are *still* burning calories and fat like crazy. Your body tends to use *fat* as fuel after an intense weight resistance routine. Building muscle is the key to a fat-burning metabolism. *Muscle is a metabolically active tissue.* This means that it burns endless calories even while you are just sitting around relaxing.

So, there you have it. Hands down, the absolute best system for taking off fat while developing strong lean muscle with no diets or starvation is: Progressive Weight Resistance, Cardio & Clean Eating.

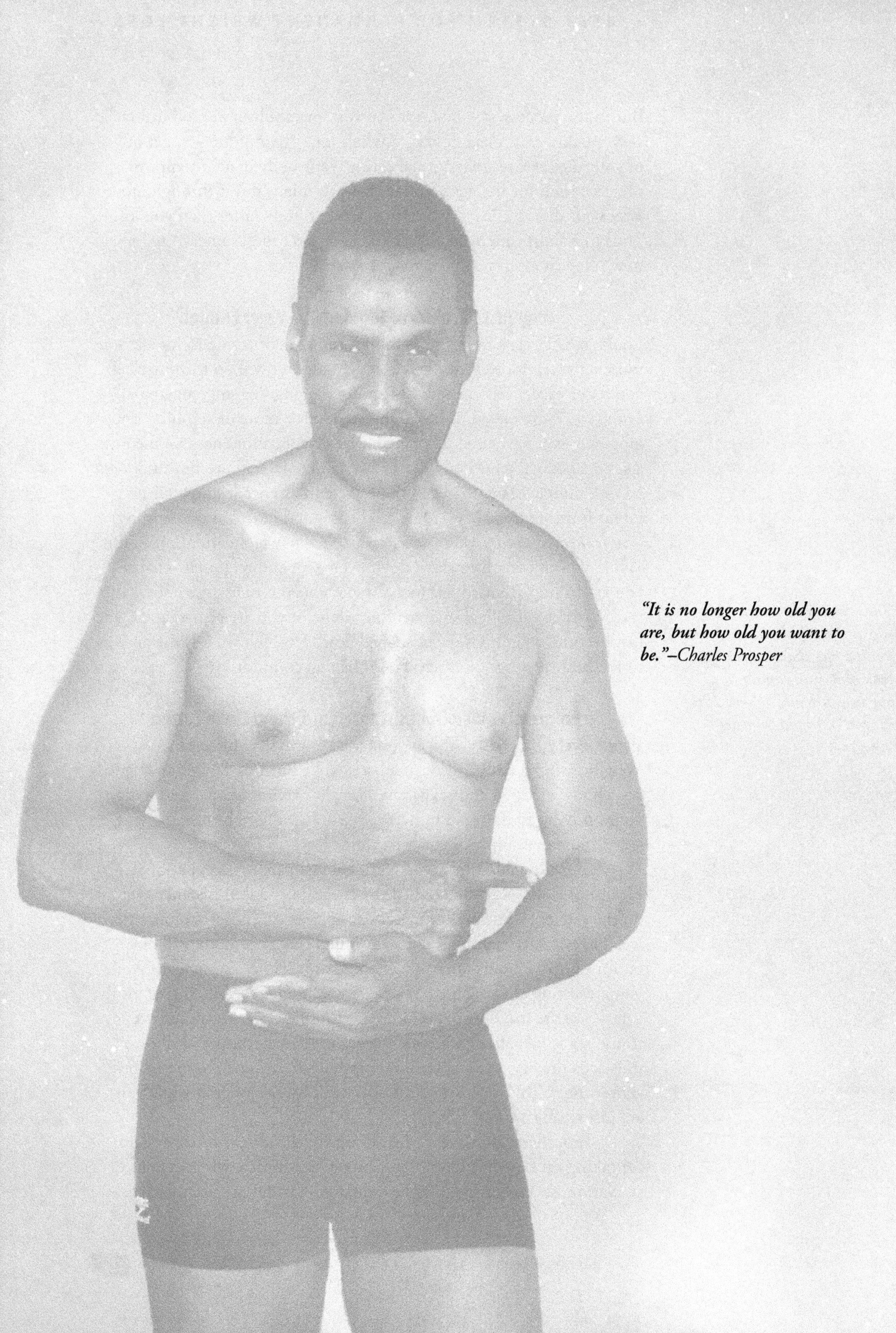

"It is no longer how old you are, but how old you want to be."–Charles Prosper

How To Eat Clean To Be Lean

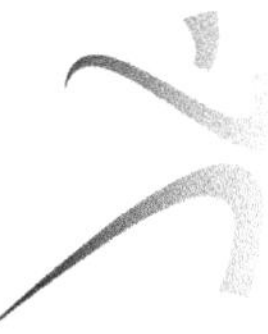

The Prosper Fit Fast System has 3 key elements: weight resistance exercise, cardio/aerobic exercise and *proper eating*. Notice, I didn't say "diet". I said proper eating – which is a whole other story. In this chapter, I will attempt to de mystify and simplify this whole puzzle of eating properly and sensibly *for the rest of your life.* It bears repeating here that diets don't work, and what I am talking about here in this chapter is a whole new life style change of clean eating habits – something that you can comfortably and happily live with. When I address health to most "baby-boomers", those currently over 50, the main concern is usually centered around that fat tire that has slowly but surely accumulated over the years. For women, it is usually about the eye-popping experience of getting into a pair of jeans that they were comfortably able to wear just 5 years ago. For the most part, and for most people, middle-age usually means a loss of muscle tone and an addition of unwanted weight. So, it is with these main concerns that I write this chapter. I will try to keep it as simple and as uncomplicated as possible.

"God eagerly awaits the chance to bless the person whose heart is turned toward Him."–Anonymous

It's All About Metabolism Control

Now I know that, already in this book, I have thrown around the word metabolism many times. Just what is our metabolism, and why is it so important? Metabolism is the amount of energy in the measurement of calories your body burns to maintain itself. Whether you are sleeping, eating, cleaning, drinking, or whatever, your body is burning calories non-stop to keep you going.

Muscle uses more calories to maintain itself than fat. People who are more muscular and have a lower percentage of body fat are said to have a higher metabolism than those who are less muscular. If you have two people who are the exact same weight and height, the one who exercises on a regular basis with weights, in addition to aerobic exercise while eating clean and healthy will have a lower percentage of body fat than the other person who never exercises, and eats fast food all of the time. The first person who exercises will have a higher metabolism than the second person who doesn't. So, what this basically means is that first person's body will use up more fat calories than the second person.

Eat One Meal A Day – Gain Weight

If you follow the typical 3 square meals a day plan of the average American diet, and should you skimp on the first two, for whatever insane reasons, and decide to "make up" and over-load on the final meal – you *will* gain weight because your metabolism slows down to conserve energy. Your body doesn't trust you. It thinks you might skip the third meal.

Eat Several Small Meals A Day – Lose Weight

Eating several small yet nutritious meals throughout the day, is a way to send a message to your body that it doesn't have to worry about your starving it. It begins to trust you by releasing fat because it has gotten to know that a regular feeding always comes every 2 or 3 hours. In other words, your metabolism speeds up.

So, How Often Should You Eat?

On the Prosper Fit Fast Program, you will eat 5 small meals per day, that is, you will eat approximately every 3 hours. Essentially, you will have three main, sit-down, *primary* meals, and there will be two *snack* meals that will fall in between. Eating like this, with this type of regularity, you will never get hungry, and most importantly, your body will not deposit extra calories as body fat. Your muscles will be bathing at practically every moment of the day in rich muscle-building amino acids and other healthy nutrients. (Amino acids are the building blocks of proteins; muscle is protein. Amino acids band together in chains to form the muscle, skin and hair, the basic stuff of which your body is made.)

"Any man can get what he desires provided he's willing to pay whatever price."–Arnold Schwarzenegger

How Many Calories Should You Eat Per Day?

Though I do not advocate the obsessive counting of calories, it is not a bad idea to keep a tab of the calories that you take in per meal in the beginning just to create a greater awareness of how many calories are in meals. After a while, with a little practice, you will not need to count calories because you know what to eat and in what proportions. You will have become a visual expert on caloric intake. But, yes, I know, I haven't answered the question. How many calories should you take in per day?

Your body can only handle about 600 calories per meal – anything over that tends to be stored away as fat. This means that if you skip breakfast and skimp on lunch, then eat a dinner feast of 3000 calories to "make up", you will have the luxury of carrying around those extra 2500 calories as *fat*. Your total daily caloric intake of roughly 2500 calories coupled with fat-burning, metabolic enhancing weight-training exercises, will melt that adipose tissue off of your body like snow sitting on a stove.

Skip Breakfast – Get Fatter

Skip breakfast, or any major meal for that matter, and your blood sugar will drop. Your appetite is triggered. Cravings follow. Then, as a survival mechanism-reaction, your thyroid and your metabolism slows. (Your thyroid and the hormones it releases play an integral part in the regulation of fat metabolism in the body.) And as I have stated many times throughout, when your metabolism slows down, you are in the fat storage mode. The food that you eat in this state, especially if it is high-caloric – *will* make you fat.

Tips and Tricks for Guaranteed Fat-Burning

Here are some of my secrets for rapid fat loss.

"You may be disappointed if you fail, but you are doomed if you don't try ."–Beverly Sills

- *Don't Eat After 8:00 p.m.* I learned this trick from a professional bodybuilder who competed and won Mr. Texas. The closer you eat to bed time, the more you are encouraging fat storage during the night. What do you think all of those extra calories are doing while you sleep? Yes, that's right. They are being stored. You must admit that sleeping is not quite a physically demanding sport.

- *Go To Bed A "Little" Hungry* I'm not talking about having skipped any of your five meals during the day. You just tend to get a little hungry every three hours. This is what your body has gotten used to. But this does not mean that you should have a meal then go to sleep. To the contrary, going to be a "little" hungry will guarantee that you will be in the fat-burning mode when you wake up.

- *Exercise Before Breakfast* If you get up and have a couple cups of water and maybe a cup of coffee then go out directly and workout, you will be burning fat like there is no tomorrow. This is the *best* time of day to exercise and burn fat. (If you do have breakfast, you should wait at least an hour and a half or two hours before your exercise.) It takes about two to three hours for food to digest and leave your stomach. If you exercise too soon, before your food has had a chance to digest properly, you may feel a little queasy and maybe want to throw up. Empty is better.

You will see fat melt like snow sitting on a stove.

The Divine Trinity of Healthy Eating

As I promised you in the beginning, I will attempt to lay out your eating guideline success as simple as possible. Before you prepare your first meal, you must understand the concept of the Divine Trinity of Eating. Actually, there is one more element (healthy fats), but I will talk about that also briefly in a moment.

The Divine Trinity of Eating:

- Protein
- Carbohydrates
- Vegetables, Salads and Fruit

The Importance of Protein

"Proscrastination is the thief of time."–Edward Young

What are proteins? Protein is the main component of your muscle tissue. This is why it is first and foremost important to promote your muscular development, increase your strength and improve your ability to handle heavier and heavier weights. You need to supply your body with ample quality protein or no growth will occur in the muscles. Proteins are your building blocks of muscular growth. There should always be plenty of protein on your plate. Now, I admit, telling you that there should be "plenty" does really help you to understand what plenty means. Here is an easy formula. Open up the palm of your hand, fingers extended outward. Good. Now imagine that you have cut off all of your fingers and thumb, and are left with just the fleshy part of your palm. *This* is approximately the portion size of protein that should be on your plate - the size of your hand, your palm, without the fingers.

Another thing about eating protein is that you should have *some* protein as a part of each of your 5 small daily meals, and you should always eat your protein first. Eating protein first slows down the absorption of the complex and or simple sugars that you might have on your plate in the form of, say, yams or dates. The problem with sugars when it hits an empty stomach is that it breaks down too fast and it is then easily converted to fat cells if you are not careful. Eating your protein first helps you to circumvent this problem. So, even if it is a "cheat meal" day, and you have decided to devour that apple pie, be sure to eat the protein portion of your plate first. This will minimize the damage of the high fat and sugar-laden dessert.

The Importance of Carbohydrates

What are carbohydrates? Carbohydrates are your body's primary source for energy. Carbohydrates are made of sugars and starches. Your body must break down carbohydrates in order to turn them into *glucose* which is commonly referred to as *blood sugar*.

There are two types of carbohydrates (called "carbs" for short in the health and fitness circles.)

- Simple Carbohydrates These are table sugar, honey, and candy which, when eaten, will give your body a quick energy surge. Then there is the energy crash where your body is let in a state of shock and jittery nerves because this type of sugar breaks down so fast in your body that it triggers an insulin spike and a consequent fat storage reaction. Too many simple carbohydrates are considered "bad" carbs and in the long run are pernicious to your health.

- Complex Carbohydrates Complex carbohydrates are made up of starchy and fiber-rich foods. These carbohydrates are processed by your digestive system much more slowly than the simple carbohydrates. When we talk about complex carbohydrates, we are talking about foods like potatoes, yams, legumes, whole wheat, beans, grains, brown rice, corn and other vegetables. Complex carbohydrates are high in nutrients. They contain plenty of vitamins, minerals, and fiber. Complex carbs leave you feeling more satiated and feel fuller longer than simple carbs. The reason for this is because they are also high fiber foods which are absorbed at a slower rate than simple carbs. Complex carbohydrates are the "good guys" of the carbohydrate world. And how much of carbohydrates should you eat? Thinking about your three *primary* meals of your, i.e, breakfast, lunch and dinner, the portion of carbohydrates on your plate should be the size of your *closed fist*.

"Chance does nothing that has not been prepared beforehand."*–Alexis de Tocqueville*

The Importance of Vegetables, Salads and Fruit

This is the third part of your Divine Food Trinity of Health. As for fresh vegetables, salads and fruit, eat as much as you wish. Vegetables form the last third of what should be on your plate. The other two thirds are protein and carbohydrates. Because they are no-fat, low-calorie and high in fiber, it is virtually impossible to overeat fresh vegetables, salads and fruit. Once you eat enough, the fiber content of it will expand in your stomach giving you a full and satisfied feeling. And you simply won't want to eat anymore.

How To Dress A Salad (Which Dressings To Avoid)

Stay away from traditional dressings like ranch and french dressing. These dressings contain way more that the regulation 20% calories from fat requirements to stay lean. Most of these dressings contain 90 to 100 of its calories from fat. The lean low-fat alternative to the traditional high-fat dressing would be:

- balsamic vinegar
- flaxseed oil
- virgin olive oil
- lemon juice (and a pinch of salt)

You can combine the above ingredients in creative ways. You can mix flaxseed oil with the balsamic vinegar (and a pinch of salt), virgin olive oil with lemon juice or balsamic vinegar and olive oil. You know what? Last night I ate a fresh garden salad with just a pinch of salt – and it tasted just great! How about that!

"Experience is the best teacher, after you have read and studied it in a book."–Charles Prosper

You Need Some "Good Fats" In Your Diet

Though we want to eliminate or mininize the intake of artery-clogging, bad, greasy fats that we find in fried food from our diets, we still need to have some "good fats" as part of our diet. If we eliminate *all* fats from our diet, our hair would fall out and our skin would crack and peel. Good fats are the lubricants of our cells and of a healthy metabolism.

Good Fats	**Bad Fats**
• raw nuts	• fried chicken
• almonds	• french fries
• cashews	• fried eggs over easy
• walnuts	• fried zucchini
• pecans	• egg rolls
• flaxseed oil	• potato chips
• avocadoes	• greasy hamburgers
• virgin olive oil	• mayonnaise
• salmon	• lard
• omega-3 fish oil	• fried onion rings

This is not an all-inclusive list, but I think you get the idea. Notice that the operant word for bad fats centers around anything that is fried.

And How Much "Good Fats" Should I Consume?

You don't need to take in too much "good fats". For example, just take a tablespoon or two of flaxseed oil (obtainable at any health food store) or the same of virgin olive oil, and add it to your vegetable or salads, and your need for your daily good fats are taken care of. An alternative to flaxseed oil or olive oil are nuts, seeds and avocados. A small handful of raw nuts at a mid-morning or mid-afternoon snack will do the trick. You can also add fresh avocado to a noon-time salad for a dose of healthy fats or if you happen to prepare some baked salmon, you've got both high quality protein and healthy Omega-3 fats. (Omega-3 fats are considered essential fatty acids. They are essential to human health and cannot be manufactured by the body therefore they must be obtained from food. Omega-3 fatty acids are highly concentrated in the brain and appear to be particularly important for cognitive brain memory and performance. Clinical studies suggests that Omega-3 fatty acid intake (especially from fish) helps protect against stroke caused by plaque buildup and blood clots in the arteries that lead to the brain.)

Nuts Are Great (But Raw Only)

"Men don't fail, they only stop trying."–Anonymous

The natural good fats and protein that you get from raw nuts, like almonds, cashews, walnuts and pecans are great (only a small handful at a time, please). However, the minute you opt for roasted and/or salted nuts, you've begun to lose it's original value. The moment you heat up any naturally occurring fat or oil, healthy fat now begins to turn into bad fat. This is like taking one of the best "good fats" around, like flaxseed oil and frying a fish with it. That good fat has now become a bad fat.

The Four Rules of Healthy Cooking and Food Preparation

- Baked not fried
- Low sugar or no sugar (Splenda instead)
- Low butter or no butter (Pam instead)
- Low cooking oil or no cooking oil (Pam instead)

When it comes to preparing and eating ***vegetables***, the rules are simple:

- *Avoid* soggy, canned vegetables.
- Fresh, uncooked is best. Flash frozen is next best.

Avoid preparing your food with oil or butter. This should be used sparingly or not at all. Hold the mayo!

You should always steam, bake, grill or broil your food. Don't fry your food, and don't even *think* about using artery-clogging lard or bacon fat. Yuck!!

What About Fruit?

Fruit. Yummy. Nature's dessert. Just include a small serving of low-calorie fruit with two or three of your primary meals, say, lunch or dinner as a dessert. Wait! How about a tasty scoop of non-fat lemon sorbet with fresh strawberries on top for lunch or dinner? A nice and tasty treat to say the least.

On the following pages, let's take a look at some healthy selection combination possibilities with Proteins, Carbohydrates and Vegetables and Fruit. And let's see what a 5-day meal plan would look like. One is filled out as a sample, and another is left blank for you to photocopy and create your own 5-day meal planner notebook.

"The deed is everything, the glory nothing."–Johann Wolfang von Goethe

Prosper
–Fit Fast–
System

Fit Fast Food Planner

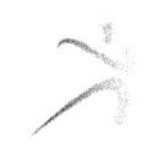

Protein	Carbhydrates	Vegetables
egg whites	yams	asparagus
turkey breast	brown rice	broccoli
tuna	grits	spinach
chicken breast	sweet potatoes	bell peppers
shrimp	black beans	lettuce
non-fat cottage cheese	corn on the cob	cauliflower
crab	green peas	cabbage
lean ground beef	lentils	carrots
orange roughy fish	red beans	celery
red snapper fish	white beans	brussels sprouts
salmon	oatmeal	wild onion
sole	Cream of Wheat	garlic
haddock	black eye peas	artichoke
mahi-mahi	baked potato	mushrooms
scallops	non-fat yogurt	cucumbers
lobster	whole-wheat bread	zucchini
soy beans	oranges	squash
protein powder	apples	parsley
top sirloin steak	berries	green beans

Make a meal with one from the protein column and one from the carb column. Now add a serving of vegetables with at least two of your five meals.

Prosper
–Fit Fast–
System

5-Meal-A-Day Planner

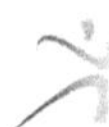

Date: 2/18/10	Day: Thursday
Total protein portions: 5	Total protein portions: 5
Total carbs portions: 5	Total carbs portions: 5

PLAN		ACTUAL	
Breakfast	4 scrambled egg whites	**Breakfast**	4 scrambled egg whites
7:00 ☑ a.m.	bowl of hot oatmeal	7:35 ☑ a.m.	bowl of hot oatmeal
☐ p.m.	1/2 banana	☐ p.m.	1/2 banana
	2 cups of water		2 cups of water
Mid-Morning	protein powder & skim milk	**Mid-Morning**	protein powder & skim milk
10:00 ☑ a.m.	handful of almonds	10:10 ☑ a.m.	handful of almonds
☐ p.m.	1 cup of green tea	☐ p.m.	1 cup of green tea
	2 cups of water		2 cups of water
Lunch	broiled chicken breast	**Lunch**	broiled chicken breast
12:00 ☐ a.m.	green salad with flaxseed oil	12:05 ☐ a.m.	green salad with flaxseed oil
☑ p.m.	fresh blueberries	☑ p.m.	fresh blueberries
	2 cups of water		2 cups of water
Mid-Afternoon	1 cup non-fat cottage cheese	**Mid-Afternoon**	1 cup non-fat cottage cheese
3:00 ☐ a.m.	3 large dates	3:15 ☐ a.m.	3 large dates
☑ p.m.	1 cup of coffee	☑ p.m.	1 cup of coffee
	2 cups of water		2 cups of water
Dinner	grilled salmon	**Dinner**	grilled salmon
6:00 ☐ a.m.	steamed vegetables	6:30 ☐ a.m.	steamed vegetables
☑ p.m.	strawberries with lemon sorbet	☑ p.m.	strawberries with lemon sorbet
	2 cups of water		2 cups of water

NOTES

I didn't feel hungry at all.

Eating like this gives me more energy.

Important: Drink 2 cups of water with each meal. Total 10 cups daily. (You may occasionally add flavored, Splenda-sweetended, no calorie Cystal Light to your water.) Taking vitamin and mineral supplements with meals is recommended though not absolutely necessary.

Prosper
–Fit Fast–
System

5-Meal-A-Day Planner

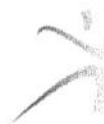

Date:	Day:
Total protein portions: 5	Total protein portions:
Total carbs portions: 5	Total carbs portions:

PLAN		ACTUAL	
Breakfast		**Breakfast**	
☑ a.m.		☑ a.m.	
☐ p.m.		☐ p.m.	
Mid-Morning		**Mid-Morning**	
☑ a.m.		☑ a.m.	
☐ p.m.		☐ p.m.	
Lunch		**Lunch**	
☐ a.m.		☐ a.m.	
☑ p.m.		☑ p.m.	
Mid-Afternoon		**Mid-Afternoon**	
☐ a.m.		☐ a.m.	
☑ p.m.		☑ p.m.	
Dinner		**Dinner**	
☐ a.m.		☐ a.m.	
☑ p.m.		☑ p.m.	

NOTES

Important: Drink 2 cups of water with each meal. Total 10 cups daily. (You may occasionally add flavored, Splenda-sweetended, no calorie Cystal Light to your water.) Taking vitamin and mineral supplements with meals is recommended though not absolutely necessary.

Let's Talk Some More About Protein

As your protein intake is of such profound importance and the cornerstone of your success, I would like to expound on it a bit more.

Remember, you should always have protein as part of every meal, and you should eat your protein before any type of dessert. By eating protein with complex carbohydrates, you slow down the speed with which *carbohydrates alone* would begin to convert into fat.

Egg Whites Are Low-Fat Protein-Delights

Take 4 eggs. (I have seen some health authors say take 8 or 10 eggs; this has always seemed a bit much for me, but you can experiment with more if you like.) The point is, that you take 4 eggs, crack them and pour just the *whites* in a bowl, being careful to keep the yolks out. (Yolks are bad news; they are fat and cholesterol city.) Scramble the egg whites briskly, add a little pepper and a pinch of salt to taste. (Take it easy with the salt.) Spray some low-fat, non-stick Pam into a frying pan and whip up some scrambled protein delights.

Milk Is Great Protein (Non-Fat Only, Please)

"Do not look to God to do something that you are not willing to do for yourself."– Charles Prosper

For what you are trying to achieve in the way of high-quality protein, milk is great for added portions of protein, but make sure it's *non-fat*. (Non-fat milk works also good with coffee, and I like Splenda as a great no-calorie sweetener.)

Tuna Is Terrific and Packed With Protein

Solid white albacore tuna packed in water is a high-quality source of low-fat protein. Just don't mess it up by adding high-fat mayo. Try the low-fat mayo version, and the caveat is - use it *sparingly!* Some eat just the tuna on a pile of fresh crisp lettuce with a little fresh lemon squeezed on the top. (My mouth is beginning to water already.)

For A-1 Protein, Broiled Chicken, Fish or Turkey Are of the Best

Broil, don't fry your protein. With fried chicken or fried fish, you have compromised the high protein value for the excess of bad fat that you must ingest along with it. And even when you broil your protein, *remove the skin*, for this is just nothing but fat that you don't need.

Whey Protein Powder for Mid-Morning or Mid-Afternoon Meals

At almost any nutrition store, you can find many quality brands of high quality whey protein powder in flavors such as chocolate, strawberry and vanilla which you can mix with non-fat cow's milk or soy milk *(for the lactose intolerant)*. Look for one that has at least 23 grams of protein with less than 20% of the calories from fat. (More on the percentage of calories from fat later.) Whey protein and a handful of nuts is a great meal.

Stay Away From Pork, Beef and Lamb

If you noticed, I didn't make much mention of beef, pork or lamb. These cuts of meat tend to be high in fat, and they are best avoided as much as possible. By comparison, there are some *relatively* healthier cuts of meat such as beef. These cuts are the top sirloin and tenderloin. Should you decide to indulge in a little beef, may I suggest that you do it on your cheat day. A little spaghetti and meatballs (easy on the sauce) is okay every now and then, but don't overdo the pasta. Healthy-wise, pasta is great, especially if you opt for the whole wheat variety – just don't pour on goo-gobs of marinara sauce.

Life is all about choices, and I think that life has provided us with enough good alternatives for every bad choice. Let's take a look and see what that means with good and poor food choices.

"It is easier to resist at the beginning than at the end."–Leonardo da Vinci

Fat Gaining Foods	Healthy Substitute Foods
• candy bar	• medjool dates
• potato chips	• baked potato chips
• hamburger	• veggie burger
• glaze donut	• whole wheat bagel (sugar-free preserves)
• peanuts	• almonds (raw)
• cheetoes	• rice cakes
• chocolate ice cream	• fat-free chocolate sorbet
• cheese nachos	• low-fat tortilla chips with fresh salsa
• corn muffin	• whole grain English muffin
• oil-popped popcorn	• air-popped popcorn

This list is not inclusive nor complete with all of the possibilities by the stretch of anyone's imagination, but you can see here that with just a little thought and a little research in all of the wonderful books out there, that deal exclusively with low-fat, high-nutrition eating, that you can most definitely find a healthy, tasty and satisfying alternative to any fast food or junk food to which you had gotten accustomed.

What Would A Typical Day of Healthy-Eating Look Like?

As you already know, you will be eating 5 small meals a day, spread out in 3 hour intervals. Just for the fun of it, let's walk through the experience of a typical healthy-eating day.

Breakfast

You should never skip breakfast. Upon awakening, your heart rate accelerates and your metabolism speeds up, making you hungry. If you take the time to have a good, nutritious and healthy breakfast, like warm oatmeal sprinkled with Splenda, a natural no-calorie sugar substitute with a little cinnamon and half a banana along with a scoop of non-fat cottage cheese and then a tablespoon of flaxseed oil, you will be *guaranteed* high energy levels all morning. Because I am lactose intolerant, I use low-fat soy milk on my oatmeal; if you're okay with non-fat skim milk, you might add a little on top. And don't forget to have 2 cups of water before leaving the table. Now, you are ready to go and take on the day. Instead of the cottage cheese mentioned above, you can also eat 4 egg whites scrambled with low-fat Pam cooking spray. (By the way, if you are eating cereal with cartoons or monsters on the box, you are watching *way* too much Saturday morning kids' shows! Stay away from all sugary-sweet dry cereals – too much sugar and fat!)

"If you don't have what you want, you are not committed to it 100%." *–Anonymous*

3-Hours Later – The Mid-Morning Meal

About 3 hours after you have had your breakfast, you schedule your mid-morning meal. It just doesn't have to be enormous, just remember that whatever you put into your mouth is a meal, and make sure that, every meal no matter how small, has a portion of protein to accompany whatever else you have on the plate. For a sample *mid-morning* meal, try:

- 1 cup of fat-free cottage cheese
- 1 small hand-full of almonds or pecans
- 1/2 apple
- 1 cup of coffee or green tea
- 2 cups of water

3-Hours Later – The Lunch Meal

Around noon-time, twelve o'clock, you are ready to enjoy your *lunch* which is considered one of your three primary meals; the other two primary meals are of course breakfast and dinner. Breakfast and dinner are interspersed with your two mini-meals: mid-morning and mid-afternoon.

Let's take a look at a typical healthy lunch.

- 1 broiled chicken breast
- 1 baked potato (no butter or sour cream)
- fresh spinach and lettuce salad (with lemon and salt)
- 1 small granola bar (for dessert)
- 2 cups of water

3-Hours Later – The Mid-Afternoon Meal

Somewhere around 3 or 4 p.m., you take out your mid-afternoon meal. This mid-afternoon, pre-dinner meal could be as simple as eating a nutritionally complete protein bar with at least 32 grams of protein and drink 2 cups of water.

Now be careful with these mega-protein bars, though they are high in protein, they are also usually high in protein *and* calories, some as high as 300 and 500 calories. Remember you want to keep each meal between 500 and 600 calories at most. If you decide to have a high protein bar as your meal, make it just that and nothing else but water. Your next meal will be dinner.

"If you are not leaning, no one will ever let you down." – *Anonymous*

In addition to the possibility of having a protein bar for this mid-afternoon snack, you could also have a glass of whey powder protein mixed in a glass of non-fat cow's milk or non-fat soy milk. You can find many good whey protein powders at your local health and nutrition store. Ask for a recommendation of a good whey powder protein with *at least* 23 grams of protein. Most of the good brands of whey protein powders found in health and nutrition stores have a low fat calorie percentage (under 20%) which is good. The nice thing about whey protein powders is that you can get them in your favorite flavors: chocolate, vanilla, banana and strawberry.

What About Drinking Water?

The rule for drinking water is quite simple – Drink 2 cups of water with each of your five health meals per day which would give you a minimum of 10 cups per day. Drinking water is very important to a healthy fat-burning metabolism. As you burn and melt away fat, the waste matter that results swims around in your blood as toxins which the body is very eager to eliminate through the urine. Drinking more water will also give you more energy as sufficient water is needed to quickly circulate the necessary nutrients to the parts of your body that your are exercising with progressive weight resistance.

Why Take Vitamin and Mineral Supplements

You *can* get all of the nutrients from your vegetables and fruit, but due to the depletion of soil minerals and overcooking a lot of our food is stripped of much of their nutrients. Take vitamin and mineral supplements with one of your *primary* meals. Here is the breakdown of a popular brand of a **Vitamin-Mineral Pack** found in health food stores.

"If you stick your head in the sand, one thing is for sure, you will get your ass kicked."–Anonymous

Supplement Facts

Serving Size: 2 Tablets

Servings per Container: 45

	Serving Amount	% DV
Vitamin A (100% as Beta Carotene)	10,000 IU	200%
Vitamin C (as Ascorbic Acid)	300 mg	500%
Vitamin D (100% as Cholecalciferol)	200 IU	50%
Vitamin E (100% as d-alpha Tocopheryl Acetate)	100 IU	333%
Vitamin K (as Phytonadione)	75 mcg	94%
Thiamin (Thiamin Mononitrate, B1)	30 mg	2000%
Riboflavin (Vitamin B2)	30 mg	1765%
Niacin (as Niacinamide)	30 mg	150%
Vitamin B6 (as Pyridoxine HCl)	30 mg	1500%
Folic Acid	400 mcg	100%
Vitamin B12 (as Cyanocobalamin)	30 mcg	500%
Biotin	250 mcg	83%
Pantothenic Acid (as d-Calcium Pantothenate)	30 mg	300%
Calcium (as Calcium Citrate)	200 mg	20%
Iodine (as Potassium Iodide)	150 mcg	100%
Magnesium (as Magnesium Oxide)	100 mg	25%
Zinc (as Zinc Oxide)	25 mg	167%
Selenium (as Selenium Yeast)	100 mcg	143%

*** Daily Value (DV) not established.*

This is quite a mouthful of vitamins and minerals that are included! And what's with all the weird abbreviations and annotations like IU, mg, mcg, DV. Throwing these words around on label really makes a pharmaceutical company feel really cool. But does the average consumer really know what they mean? And do you *really* understand what each vitamin and mineral will do for you? Let me take the trouble to break it all down for you vitamin by vitamin, mineral by mineral and abbreviation by abbreviation. Okay, let's go. Let's first start with the measurements: IU, mg, mcg and then the symbol DV and explain exactly what the % is all about.

What Is % DV?

Quite simply food label list percentages are based on recommended daily intakes, that is, the recommended amount of nutrients that you should get each day. These numbers tell you the Percent Daily Value (DV) that a serving of this vitamin or mineral provides as a percentage of experts' established standards. For example, a label may show that a vitamin provides 30 % of the daily recommended amount of vitamin A. This means you still need another 70 percent of vitamin to meet the recommended goal. The % DV is based on a 2,000-calorie diet for adults older than 18.

"The biggest risk in life is not risking."–Anonymous

What Is IU?

IU is a measure unit used with certain vitamins like vitamin E: it stands for International Units. The scientific fancy-pants definition of IU is "a unit used to measure the activity (that is, the effect) of many vitamins and drugs". This is a convoluted way of saying that a certain number of IU's of a vitamin is expected to produce a certain level of beneficial effect, be it better cardiovascular, mental or prostate health in the case of a man. More important than trying to get your head around the concept of IU measurements would be to see the % DV and make sure that you are getting 100% of whatever the value or benefit the vitamin or food stuff is supposed to afford.

What Is *mg* and *mcg*?

Well, let's start with a gram. A gram is a metric unit of weight. *mg* is a milligram. 1000 milligrams (mgs) = 1 gram. *mcg* is a microgram. 1000 micrograms = 1 milligram. For practical purposes, all you need to know that it is a measurement, a tiny one at that, based on weight. More important to know is what percentage of the total 100% recommended amounts you are getting. If you are getting 100%, *who cares* how much it weighs milligram or microgram-wise!

When you look at a vitamin supplement, wouldn't you always like to remember exactly what it is suppose to do for you? Fair enough.

Let's take a look at it and briefly explain the benefits of each of the vitamins and mineral of the previously shown vitamin/mineral label, so, the next time that you see a mega-vitamin pack you are thinking of purchasing, at least you will understand the benefits and value of each.

Vitamin A (Beta Carotene)

Beta Carotene comes from these cool colored molecules that are synthesized only in plants which show vitamin A activity. Notice that I am not saying that this is the synthetic vitamin A that you have since years past been used to. Beta carotene is closely related to vitamin A, but there is a big difference. Large doses of vitamin A definitely can cause health problems. Symptoms of a vitamin A overdose include tiredness, discomfort, lethargy, upset stomach, decreased appetite, vomiting, slow or decreased growth, joint soreness, irritability, headache, drying and cracking of the lips and skin, hair loss, and yellowing of the skin. Whoa! Not good.

Hundreds of different carotenoids are synthesized by plants, but only about 10 % of them are provitamin A carotenoids.

"Others can stop you temporarily, but only you can do it permanently."–Anonymous

The Benefits of Beta Carotene

- helps prevent night blindness
- helps eye problems
- helps skin disorders
- enhances immunity
- protects against toxins
- protects against colds, flu, and infections
- has potential to prevent and treat lung cancer
- has been shown to reduce the risk of cataracts
- it is an antioxidant protecting cells and slowing aging

Now, when you read all of these exciting and wonderful benefits, you may think, "Charles, where did you get all of this information? I am sure that you just didn't make it up." Fair question. On the following page are my references for these facts.

References

1. **Mathews-Roth MM.** *Systemic Photoprotection.* Dermatol Clinics. 1986;4:335-39

2. **Omaye ST, et al.** *Beta carotene: friend or foe.* Fundam Appl Toxicol. Dr Joseph Malak 1997;40:163-74

3. **Nishino H.** *Cancer prevention by natural carotenoids.* J Cell Biochem Suppl. 1997;27:86-91

4. **Mangles AR, et al.** *Carotenoid content of fruits and vegetables: an evaluation of analytic data.* JADA. 1993;93:284-296

5. **Gonzalez S, et al.** *Topical or oral administration with an extract of Polypodium leucotomos prevents acute sunburn.* Photodermatol Photoimmunol Photomed. 1997;13:50-60

Vitamin C (Ascorbic Acid)

"What we Are is God's gift to us. What we Become is our gift to God."–Robert Anthony

Vitamin C is also known as, ascorbic acid, dehydroascorbic acid, L-ascorbic acid and Vitamin C (L-ascorbic acid). Vitamin C cannot be manufactured by the body, so needs to be ingested daily, and it is difficult to overdose with vitamin C because ascorbic acid is a water-soluble vitamin. Toxic levels are not built up or stored in the body, and any excess is lost through the urine.

The Benefits of Vitamin C

- protects the body against pollutants
- helps prevent cataracts
- contributes to cardiovascular health
- prevents cell degeneration and premature aging
- helps to prevent skin wrinkles
- strengthens the walls of the capillary blood vessels
- promotes healthy cell development
- enhances normal tissue growth and repair

- helps in the healing of wounds and burns
- evidence shows that it may help to reduce cholesterol

Important Disclaimer

I just realized something. Some of you may use these guidelines as a substitute for seeing your doctor for any serious medical conditions. So, before we go any further to protect my arse, let me issue you this caveat.

> This information about the value and benefits of vitamins and minerals is based on reputable scientific research and, but please, this should not be for self-diagnosis or self-treatment of any disease. Always consult a medical professional regarding any medical problems and before undertaking any major dietary changes. Again, this information is not meant to be substituted for medical advice.

Okay with that understanding, let us continue.

"When love and skill work together, expect a masterpiece."–John Ruskin

Vitamin D (Cholecalciferol)

Vitamin D (Cholecalciferol) is a fat soluble vitamin often also called the sunshine vitamin because the ultraviolet B rays of the sun cause skin oils to produce this vitamin. Fair-skinned people get the recommended daily dose of Vitamin D with 30 minutes of sunlight exposure twice a week while darker-skinned people require longer exposures for the light to penetrate the skin. Excessive exposure to the sun will not result in an overdose of Vitamin D, because the body will simply stop the production and conversion of this vitamin as soon as it reaches the level that it needs. The body's ability to manufacture Vitamin D declines with age. Older people and people who don't go outside and get sun that much may become deficient in this vitamin. Vitamin D amongst other things is important in its role of making phosphorus and calcium available for the body.

The RDA for Vitamin D is 400 IU a day (200 IU for children, 600 IU for over age 70). Vitamin D is the most toxic of all vitamins, therefore avoid supplementing doses more than twice the recommended daily dose for children or more than 10 times the recommended daily dose for adults. Vitamin D toxicity can produce constipation or diarrhea, headache, appetite loss, nausea, vomiting, irregular heartbeat, and fatigue. So, take the recommended daily dose of 400 IU a day for adults and 200 IU for children. If you are 70 or older, 600 IU is okay.

The Benefits of Vitamin D

- promotes healthy bones and strong teeth
- helps the absorption calcium and phosphorus
- prevents rickets in children
- may help prevent colon, breast, and prostate cancer
- prevents osteomalacia in adults
- helps prevent osteoporosis

Vitamin E (d-alpha Tocopherol Acetate)

Tocopherols (or TCP) are a class of chemical compounds of which many have vitamin E activity. Vitamin E deficiency causes neurological problems due to poor nerve conduction. Deficiency can also cause anemia, due to oxidative damage to red blood cells.

"Luck is believing you're lucky."–Tennessee Williams

The Benefits of Vitamin E

- helps in the prevention of cataracts
- helps in the prevention of glaucoma
- helps in the prevention of heart disease
- may help prevent Parkinson's disease
- contributes to mental health
- promotes prostate health
- promotes healthy joints
- promote healthy skin, hair and eyes

Vitamin K (Phytonadione)

Vitamin K? Most people have never heard of this one. Let's see what vitamin K is all about. Vitamin K, otherwise known as phytonadione, promotes healthy normal blood clotting. Great sources of this vitamin include dark leafy greens, broccoli, spinach, seaweed, turnip greens, asparagus, cabbage, alfalfa, green leafy lettuce and cheddar cheese. Symptoms of deficiency of vitamin K include a prolonged clotting time, easy bleeding, and bruising. This deficiency is uncommon in adults and it is usually limited to people who have problems with liver or food absorption disorders.

Recommended doses of vitamin K are:

- **For Men**: 80 mcg
- **For Women**: 65 mcg.

(mcg is micrograms in case you have forgotten.)

The Benefits of Vitamin K

- promotes healthy kidney functioning
- promotes normal growth and development
- regulates normal blood clotting

"If you would have a faithful servant, and one that you like, serve yourself."–Benjamin Franklin

Vitamin B1 (Thiamin Mononitrate)

Thiamin (also spelled "thiamine") is a water-soluble B-complex vitamin. It is also known as vitamin B1 or aneurine. Thiamin is involved in nervous system and muscle functioning, enzyme processes, breakdown of carbohydrates and production of hydrochloric acid (which is needed for digestion). There is very little thiamin stored in the body, and depletion can occur quickly. Severe chronic thiamin deficiency can cause potentially serious complications involving the nervous system/brain, muscles.

Vitamin B1, or thiamin, is one of 8 B vitamins. All B vitamins help the body to convert food (carbohydrates) into fuel (glucose), which is "burned" to produce energy. These B vitamins, often referred to as B complex vitamins, also help the body metabolize fats and protein.

The Benefits of Vitamin B1 (Thiamin)

- promotes healthy skin
- promotes healthy eyes
- promotes healthy hair

- promotes a healthy liver
- helps the nervous system function properly
- improves the body's ability to withstand stress

Thiamin was so named B1 because it was the first B vitamin to be discovered.

Vitamin B2 (Riboflavin)

Vitamin B2, a water-soluble vitamin, is also called riboflavin, works with other vitamins in the B complex to process calories from carbohydrates, protein and fat. If water-soluble vitamins are not used by the body, they are eliminated in the urine; this means that you need a continuous supply of water-soluble vitamins such as vitamin B2 (Riboflavin) in your food. Riboflavin is absorbed into the bloodstream through the walls of the small intestine. It is carried to the tissues of the body and incorporated into the cell enzymes. The liver is the major site of storage. It contains about one-third of the total riboflavin in the body.

The liver, heart and kidneys have the richest concentrations of this vitamin. Riboflavin is found naturally in green leafy vegetables, riboflavin-enriched breads and cereal, red meats and diary products. However the body does not store large quantities of vitamin B2 so to make sure, it is great to take it as part of your supplementary diet.

"Trust in God and do something."–Mary Lyon

The Benefits of Vitamin B2 (Riboflavin)

- promotes healthy skin and good vision
- promotes growth red cell production
- aides in your digestion of food
- helps in the functioning of the nervous system
- helps to prevent constipation
- promotes healthy nails
- promotes healthy hair
- strengthens mucous lining of mouth, lips, and tongue
- alleviates eye strain

Niacin - Vitamin B3 (Niacinamide)

Vitamin B-3 (Niacin) is also known as niacinamide, and is one of the water-soluble B-complex vitamins. Niacinamide was first linked to preventing the development of diabetes in experimental animals in the 1950s, a finding confirmed in the 1980s which led to further clinical studies. Niacinamide enhances insulin secretion and increases insulin sensitivity. Evidence points to niacinamide supplements as being very effective in the preventing of type I diabetes from progressing in some patients if given soon enough at the onset of diabetes. Some natural sources of niacinamide include sunflower seeds, peanuts, tuna, turkey, chicken, halibut, brewer's yeast, beef liver, salmon, swordfish and halibut.

The Benefits of Niacin - Vitamin B3

- maintains the normal functioning of the nerves
- aides the digestive system
- maintains normal functioning of the skin
- prevents premenstrual headache
- treats dizziness and ringing in the ears
- dilates the blood vessels for better circulation
- helps to reduce high cholesterol levels

"Oh Lord, thou givest us everything at the price of effort."–Leonardo da Vinci

When you take the extended release capsules be sure to swallow them whole and not to chew or crush them, and be sure to take them with or immediately after food to decrease the possibility of stomach irritation.

Vitamin B6 (Pyridoxine HCL)

Vitamin B6 (Pyridoxine HCL) is Pyridoxine Hydrochloride This is another water-soluble vitamin of the the B-family of vitamins. Vitamin B6 is responsible for over 100 known enzyme reactions in the body. Pyridoxine HCL is mostly related to the metabolism of proteins and amino acids. B6 is found naturally in potatoes, brown rice, bananas, peanuts, brewers yeast, whole grains, legumes, wheat cream, eggs, chicken, carrots, liver and other organ meats. B6 is also found in fish. Pyridoxine HCL aides in the production of hemoglobin of red blood cells, and it aides in the production of neurotransmitters like serotonin which is important for a good night's sleep.

Vitamin B6 may be toxic in doses of 2,000 mgs or more per day, so, don't overdo it.

The Benefits of Vitamin B6 (Pyridoxine HCL)

- aides cardiovascular efficiency
- improves over-all energy production in the body
- alleviates premenstrual syndrome symptoms
- enhance cognitive performance in older adults
- may lower the risk of Alzheimer's disease
- improving nerve-related problems in diabetic patients
- helps to reduce high cholesterol levels

"To play it safe is not to play."–Robert Altman

Folic Acid

To be quite honest, before I started doing the research for this book, I always wondered what the heck is folic acid? It is amazing how we will be impressed by names of vitamins and minerals even to the point of ingesting them without having the faintest idea what some of them are for. Well, now, no more mystery around folic acid.

Guess what? *Folic acid* is really another one of the *B-Complex* vitamins. Boy, there are surely a lot of these guys. Folic acid is also known as Vitamin B9, it plays an important role in cell maintenance and repair. It aides in amino acid metabolism as well as in the formation of red and white blood cells. Folic acid can be found in fruits, green leafy vegetables and yeast.

The Benefits of Folic Acid

- it helps to inhibit colon cancer
- aides in the prevention of heart disease
- relief from depression
- helps reduce the risks of high blood pressure

Vitamin B12 (Cyanocobalamin)

Vitamin B-12 is also known as cyanocobalamin. It works as a coenzyme in the creation of your all-important DNA material. Vitamin B-12 aides in cell development growth, and it is vital to carbohydrate, fat, and protein metabolism. B-12 is not found in plant foods, however you can find cyanocobalamin in eggs, meats, fish, and dairy products.

The Benefits of Vitamin B12 (Cyanocobalamin)

- aides in healthy development of skin, hair and nerves
- metabolizes amino acids and fatty acids
- aides in healthy development of blood cells
- helps to treat Alzheimer's disease
- improves the immune system
- helps alleviate nervous disorders
- aides in the release of food energy

"My belief is God unto myself."–Charles Prosper

The recommended daily dose for men is 2.4 mcg. And the recommended daily dose for women is 2.4 mcg as well.

Biotin

Biotin is one of eight essential vitamins that comprise the B-complex. Like all of the members of the B-complex, biotin plays an important role in energy metabolism, acting as a coenzyme in chemical reactions that produce energy. Biotin is a key player in fat synthesis, amino acid metabolism and the creation of glycogen, the body's short-term energy supply that is stored in muscle. Biotin is only needed in small amounts; the intestines also may produce small amounts of biotin.

Biotin can be found naturally in food such as legumes, cauliflower, egg yolk, nuts, sardines, brewer's yeast, and kidney and liver meats.

The Benefits of Biotin

- the ability to maintain healthy shiny hair
- may help the hair keep its color longer

- benefits the treatment of muscle pain

It is recommended that you consult with your physician before taking dosages of biotin larger than 10 mg.

Pantothenic Acid (d-Calcium Pantothenate)

Panothenic Acid is also known as vitamin B5, and it is another water soluble vitamin of the vitamin B-complex family.

The Benefits of Pantothenic Acid

- accelerate wound and scar healing
- aides in the healing of acne
- helps protect the body from various toxins

Calcium (Calcium Citrate)

"Self-trust is the first secret of success."–Ralph Waldo Emerson

Over 99% of your body's calcium is in your skeleton. This is what gives your frame its important mechanical rigidity. When calcium intake is lower than normal, the skeleton is used as a reserve to meet needs. Long-term use of skeletal calcium to meet these needs leads to osteoporosis. Americans have a high risk of osteoporosis, since their average diet contains only 600 mg of calcium daily. Experts suggest the daily dose for calcium be 1,300 mg for people ages 9 to 18, 1,000 to 1,200 mg for adults 19 to 50, and 1,500 mg for people over 50. Be careful not to take too much calcium for this may cause kidney stones and interfere with iron absorption. The best way to use calcium to build bone mass and to ward off osteoporosis is to take it in addition to regular physical exercise that involves progressive weight resistance.

The Benefits of Calcium

- protects against osteoporosis
- helps to form healthy bones and teeth
- aides the transmission of nerve messages
- the proper functioning of the heart muscle
- activates important enzymes for digestion

Iodine (Potassium Iodide)

Iodine is required by humans for the synthesis of thyroid hormones. Chronic iodine deficiency can lead to numerous health problems in children and adults, including thyroid gland dysfunction and various neurologic, gastrointestinal, and skin abnormalities.

The Benefits of Iodine

- maintains a healthy thyroid
- avoids neurological disorders
- helps maintain the health of digestion

Iodine deficiency is rare in developed countries like the United States and Canada due to the enrichment of iodine in table salt.

Magnesium (Magnesium Oxide)

"Don't ask of your friends what you yourself can do."–Quintus Ennius

One of the most salient benefits of the mineral magnesium is in the development of strong bones. Magnesium is an essential supplement for many parts of the body, including the muscular and nervous systems. Magnesium has many benefits, including its ability to clean out the body.

The Benefits of Magnesium

- helps to prevent osteoporosis
- helps to alleviate hypertension
- aides in the relief of constipation
- helps in the relief of migraines

Zinc (Zinc Oxide)

Zinc is a natural mineral found in all plants and animals. The recommended daily dose of zinc is 15mg. Zinc is essential for growth. It controls our enzymes and renews the cells in our bodies. DNA is also made possible in part because of zinc. The best sources of zinc are oysters, some seafoods, lean red meats, liver, cereals, brown rice, dairy products and nuts.

The Benefits of Zinc

- helps maintain healthy vision
- promotes a healthy immune system
- accelerates the healing of wounds

Zinc is involved in the fertility in adults. Zinc increases both sperm count and sperm motility. It is important for the health of reproductive organs and the prostate gland. Isn't it curious also that in many cultures oysters are considered as an aphrodisiac? Is it a coincidence that oysters are particularly very high in zinc?

Selenium (Selenium Yeast)

Selenium is a vital mineral that works well together with vitamin E for overall health. The recommended dietary allowance (RDA) for those 11 years and older is 55 micrograms. This amount is fairly easy to get through a reasonably balanced diet. Selenium is found in seafood, lean meat, organ meats, dairy products, chicken, oatmeal, brown rice, Brazil nuts, broccoli, garlic, kelp, molasses, onions, and brewer's yeast.

"If you don't stand for something, you'll fall for anything."–Michael Evans

The Benefits of Selenium

- promotes a healthy heart
- protects against various forms of cancer
- aides the transmission of nerve messages
- helps to slow down the aging process
- helps to prevent arthritis

Take It Easy When Taking Big-Ass Vitamin Tablets

When I take my vitamin and mineral supplements, I have about 5 or 6 different containers of supplements. Why so many? Well, when manufacturers attempt to force the potency of say, 25 vitamins and minerals, all into a *couple* of tablets, you are going to have two *gi-normous*, horse-pill sized tablets that will be hard to swallow and sometimes hard to digest. With these gigantic tablets, you *have* to take them with food for better absorption. Bottom line – a mega-vitamin pack of 7 tablets is a much better digestive option than taking 2 big ones.

How To Calculate The % of Fat Calories from a Nutrition Label

I would like to show you, now, how to read a Nutrition Label so that you are always able to make the correct and healthy food choices. One of the most important things that you should learn is how to read and quickly calculate the percentage of fat calories from a Nutrition Label. This is the bottom line. You should always aim to ingest foods that contain about 20% of its calories from fat. If you are anything over 20%, you are taking in more fat calories than you want to be in the fat-burning mode. You might go up to 25% every now and then, but the goal is to stay within the parameters of 20% fat calories or less. When you stay at 20% fat calories of what you eat, no problem, you are *definitely* on the right road to burning fat. 25% fat calories is *stretching* it, but it's passable.

So, how can you quickly learn to calculate the fat calories percentage from the Nutrition Labels that you see? Well, for example, let's take a look at the Nutrition Facts that I took from the label of a popular protein-plus power bar.

"Do what you can, with what you have, where you are."– Theodore Roosevelt

Nutrition Facts Serving Size: 1 Bar (85g), Amount Per Serving: **Calories** 310, Calories from Fat 80, **Total Fat** 9g (**14**% DV), Saturated Fat 7g (37% DV), Trans Fat 0g, **Cholesterol** 5mg (2% DV), **Sodium** 230mg (9% DV), **Potassium** 270mg (**8**% DV), **Total Carbohydrate** 32g (**11**% DV), Dietary Fiber 2g (**9**% DV), Sugars 3g, Sugar Alcohol 25g, **Protein** 32g (**35**% DV), Vitamin A (30% DV), Vitamin C (30% DV), Calcium (45% DV), Iron (15% DV), Vitamin E (30% DV), Thiamin (30% DV), Riboflavin (40% DV), Niacin (30% DV), Vitamin B-6 (30% DV), Folic Acid (30% DV), Vitamin B-12 (30% DV), Biotin (30% DV), Pantothenic Acid (30% DV), Phosphorus (25% DV), Iodine (35% DV), Magnesium (15% DV), Zinc (30% DV), Copper (30% DV), Percent Daily Values (DV) are based on a 2,000 calorie diet.

Now, let's just take a look at the information here about **Total Fat** percentage. It's says (14% DV). This can be deceptive if you don't know how to read it. Just at first blush, you would think, "Wow! This is great - only 14% fat calories!" Not! They are not giving you the total calories from fat for this nutrition bar. They are telling you that this is the recommended Daily Value (DV) of fat that you have *in the entire day!* All of the DV percentages (Daily Value) is a percentage of what you are expecting to eat in the entire course of the day of a 2000 calorie diet. Now, let me show you how to always calculate the *real* percent of fat calories *for this nutrition bar*. Here are the steps:

1. Look for the **Total Calories**. In our example of this protein nutrition bar, what are the ***Total*** Calories? I want you to look at the page again and give me your answer. What did you decide? If you said *310 Calories*, I am proud of you as that is correct.

2. Look for the **Calories from Fat**. Look again and tell me the answer. Great! You got that one that time with no problem. The answer of course is *Calories from Fat 80*.

3. Large Into Small = Percent. This is your formula to get the percentage of *fat* calories of the total calories *for this nutrition bar*.

From here it is nothing but a little high school math. Remember, you are to *divide* the larger number (Total Calories) into the smaller number (Calories from Fat).

"A consciousness of God releases the greatest power of all." *–Science of Mind*

If we do this as a fraction, it will look like this:

$$\frac{80}{310} =$$

Or we can express the same division problem as:

$$80 \div 310 =$$

Or, you can simply whip out your pocket calculator.

Whether you do it by hand, in your head or with a pocket calculator, the correct percentage that you will get for this product will be – ***25% calories from fat.*** As you can see, without this formula and without this understanding, you would mistakenly be reading the DV%. This gets to be fun once you get the hang of it. After doing this with your pocket calculator a few dozen times, you will find that you will get more and more accurate, and you will be able to know what has too many calories from fat just by looking at it.

Why Does Even Junk Food Have Nutrition Fact Labels?

Pick up a bag of any obvious type of junk food that you wish – chocolate cookies, candy bars, potato chips, onion rings...your choice. You will notice something that I find very curious. All of them have a

Nutrition Facts label. But what nutrition could they be talking about? First of all, let me explain that by law, all food stuff requires a Nutrition Fact label to let the consumer know what he or she is getting. But clever marketers have upped the anty by using this regulation to their creative marketing advantage. Now, I am taking you somewhere with this, but before I do, I want to try a little experiment with you. Ready? Now, no matter what you do right now as you read these words, I do *not* want you to think of a pink elephant! Well, we all know what you are thinking about now, don't we? You see, just the mention of something forces the thought and therefore the association in your mind. When you see the *word* "**Nutrition**" **Facts**, on these labels you are thinking about this food now from the subliminal perspective of it being a "*type*" *of nutrition*. This kind of eases your conscience in eating it. But wait, there's more! – as they say on the late night T.V. infomercials. I have seen some candy labels that will say something like this:

Vitamin A	0%	•	Vitamin C	0%
Calcium	10%	•	Iron	2%
Not a Significant Source of Dietary Fiber * Percent Daily Values are based on a 2,000 calorie diet.				

"The purpose of life is a life of purpose."–*Robert Byrne*

By law, a food company is only required to indicate that which the item contains. It is *not* necessary to say what it doesn't contain, but there is no regulation which prohibits this as long as you are telling the truth. My point is this. Look at the example above. If there is no Vitamin in this product, what the point in saying **Vitamin A 0%** or saying **Vitamin C 0%?** It's just like the pink elephant I asked you not to think about. The minute they say, or rather, the minute you see, read and *think* **Vitamin A** or **Vitamin C** in association with that product – they gotcha! Even though it is 0%, you are still associating vitamin content with that product even though it doesn't exist, just by virtue of the *thought* of it on that label. "Well, those potato chips couldn't be *that* bad! At least they have **Vitamin C 0%**!" This is your unconscious, subliminal thought process.

But wait, I'm not done yet. The label is clever also in another way, that is, it's saying what it *doesn't* have for you to sort of think in a certain way it does have what it says, simply because it mentions it on the label. Check it out. "Not a Significant Source of Dietary Fiber." Most of that junk doesn't have *any* dietary fiber! So what's the point in mentioning it? Well, you will just have to imagine what "Significant" means here – and *hope* that there is enough in there that you won't wind up getting constipated in the end!

How To Eat Out (Ordering in A Restaurant)

Well, this is the real world. I can't expect for you to always prepare your food. And I surely wouldn't want you to become a recluse, refusing every dinner invitation that is presented to you. You can very well eat in restaurants. (I didn't say your typical greasy, fast food artery cloggers.) You can eat in nice restaurants. It is just a matter of tweaking what you select and how you have them prepare it.

Let me give you some practical tips for eating out:

1. Avoid going to eat out when you are *very* hungry, as you will tend to overdo it.

2. Order à la carte whenever necessary. For example, if you are at breakfast, instead of eating scrambled whole eggs, request scrambled egg whites.

3. Have your baked potatoes served without the butter or the sour cream. Chopped chives, pepper and a pinch of salt is sufficient.

"As soon as you trust yourself, you will know how to live."–Johann von Goethe

4. Skip the booze and the wine (high calories and sugar), let alone the intoxication of the alcohol itself. Sorry. Hard choices here.

5. Think grilled or baked – never fried anything. Grilled breast of chicken is yours – *not* the Southern fried chicken. Fresh steamed vegetables is what you should order – *not* the fried zucchini.

6. Dessert is fine, but think low fat. Frozen non-fat sorbet – *not* chocolate ice cream with fudge syrup. Sugary pies and cakes are always a problem. (Exception – a piece of apple pie for dessert on your "cheat" day.)

7. Stay away from carbonated sodas. One can of your favorite cola can contain more than 12 teaspoons of sugar, and let me remind you that a sugar spike in your system, especially if you are drinking a soda pop on an empty stomach, will trigger a sudden rise in your blood insulin which will tell your body to store fat. The carbonation of the soda swells and bloats the stomach. It may have been fun burping soda as a kid, but you weren't that worried about your waistline at that time. Opt for ice tea with a no-calorie sweetener.

AlwaysTake Your Lunch To Work

Be prepared. Avoid the take-out grease. Save money. Live healthier. There are plenty of reasons to avoid eating out or at least avoiding the fast-food eating habit. We are creatures of habit, and new habits once formed are blessings set on automatic.

Buy Yourself the Biggest Lunch Box You Can Find

You soon want to have the reputation at work for the person with the largest lunch box. Remember, you are preparing and carrying around, your mid-morning meal, your lunch and your mid-afternoon meal. You want to go out and find the biggest lunch box available. I remember once a co-worker said to me: "Charles, I didn't know you were moving." Implying that my lunch box was the size of a suitcase. It was big – but not *that* big!

Stay Away from Cold Cuts

Your bologna, salami, sliced ham and sliced turkey are frequently injected with lots of nasty chemicals, water and way too much sodium, i.e, salt. Opting to pack a roasted breast of chicken which you slice yourself is a much better choice. And for heavens sake, stay away from anything that is sausage. This is always bad news and an invitation to ingest a lot of bad fat and cholesterol into your heart and arteries. My mother, may she rest in peace, died from a stroke caused by clogged arteries to the brain. Cholesterol is a killer, and over time is nothing to be taken lightly - especially if you have been fortunate enough to reach and enjoy middle age.

"We pray to God that He may answer our prayer, and God prays to us that we may believe–so that we may receive that which we pray for."–Charles Prosper

Stay Away from Trans-Fat (Hydrogenated Oils)

Trans-fat repackaged as hydrogenated or partially hydrogenated oil is the most villainous, artery-clogging, cancer-causing substance that you might put into your body. Cookies, though friends to your taste buds, are mortal enemies to your body and health in that, over time, they deposit and accumulate hydrogenated fat into your body and arteries; cookies and cakes will also spike your insulin which signals your body to store fat rather than burn it. Crackers, as innocuos-looking as they are, contain nothing but bleached white flour, hydrogenated oil and lots of fat calories. Sit down and eat enough crackers on a daily, regular basis, and your will begin to wear those crackers as extra pounds on your waist, thighs and butt.

Avoid, Minimize or Eliminate Alcohol Consumption Entirely

One twelve-once beer contains about 150 calories – bad calories. These are calories which harden and clog your arteries and slow down your good fat-burning processes. During your first 12 weeks on the *Prosper Fit-Fast*

Program, I would strongly suggest that you avoid your alcohol consumption altogether. But if drink you must, select the drinks with the lowest alcohol and the lowest calorie content.

"Fat–Free" + High Sugar = Fat Storage

Just because a food says *"95% Fat-Free!"* doesn't necessarily mean that you won't get fat and gain weight. Let me explain. Let us say that you eat a "low-fat" cookie or a "low-fat" pie. So far so good. But most cookies and pies are almost always *high* in sugar! Now, this high-in-sugar part of the equation is a very critical factor. High *simple sugar* ingested into your body, and even worse if you eat them on an empty stomach, will break down *too quickly* into your bloodstream and *will* be stored as fat. High sugar levels in your blood also triggers a sudden elevation in insulin which sends a fat-storage message to your body. And we are not even taking into consideration the nervous shock and jitters all of this elevated sugar can do to your body as well as lasting sometimes for hours later.

The good news about once you begin the *Prosper Fit Fast System* is that in about 2 or 3 weeks, you will begin to lose your cravings for fat and sugar. Be patient, and trust your body. Give it a little time. It will surprise you.

"I finally figured out the only reason to be alive is to enjoy it." *–Rita Mae Brown*

In the last few sections, I went over a lot of foods and stuff that you should avoid, but what, might you ask are some of my favorite foods? There are many, but here are some that stand out.

Oatmeal Is King

Whole oats cooked on the stove is one of the best long-term energy-producing hot meals that I have ever experienced. (And you don't have to wait to eat it for breakfast. You can have it in the afternoon or evening as well.) Just sprinkle onto it a little Splenda no-calorie sweetener, a little cinnamon, half a banana and some non-fat milk (cow's or soy milk) and – Shazaam! – you have just made yourself a super-meal. If it's breakfast, you can scramble up 4 egg whites in Pam low-fat, non-stick spray. Have a slice of apple if you wish, and you will feel as though you are infused with some super powers! Don't be surprised if you fly around the room like a fly.

You can vary up your breakfast experience. Instead of oatmeal, try Cream of Wheat or grits. As always, skip the butter. (Now I am from New Orleans where it is *illegal* to eat grits without butter, so I sometimes, due to my upbringing, will put just a *teensy* bit of butter for a little flavor.) Just do the butter thing a little or not at all.

You Can't Beat Beans

Red beans, kidney beans, black beans, split peas and lentils are all wonderfully nutritious food. They have lots of fiber and good quality protein. (Soybeans are in a class of their own as they are one of the few beans that have all of the essential amino acids in the same way the meat or chicken has.) Beans and rice, a great Southern states dish of the U.S., make an excellent meal, consisting of rich and complex, energy-generating carbohydrates.

Brown Rice Rocks

Whole-grain brown rice is the way to go over eating the common-place white long grain rice. Whole-grain brown rice is far superior because it contains the important vitamin-B rich bran still intact. Whole-grain brown rice, with its slightly crunchy, nutty flavor has more important colon-cleansing fiber.

Salads , Fresh Vegetables and Fruit – Eat As Much As You Want

Fresh vegetables usually have very few calories. Vegetables are the fibrous carbohydrates which after giving your body it's necessary nutrients, will then, through the fiber it contains, sweep through your intestines collecting junk, fatty acids and nasty deposits thus leaving your intestines squeaky clean which allows you to absorb more of the vitamins and other nutrients that you are getting from all of the other healthy food you are eating.

"Our remedies oft in ourselves do lie."–William Shakespeare

You can't eat too much fruit (or fresh vegetables for that matter) because they fill you quickly because of the fiber that naturally expands in your stomach once you eat enough. Eat enough fruit or fresh vegetables, and your appetite for more will just stop naturally because of the full and satisfied feeling they give you.

As for food preparation, fresh is best. Flash frozen vegetables are the next best, and soggy, canned and lifeless vegetables are better avoided. And if you must cook, steam, not boil your veggies – the best way to go.

Now, I know that I have given you a lot of information about food choices in this chapter, but let me make things a little simpler for you by giving you a sample experience of a 6-Day Meal Plan starting with Day 1. Remember, you are eating every three hours, and one of your seven days of the week is your "cheat day" to each whatever you want.

Day One

BREAKFAST: 1/2 cup of oatmeal, 1/2 banana, 4 scrambled egg whites in Pam, coffee, 2 cups of water

MID-MORNING MEAL: 1/2 cup of non-fat yogurt, a small handful of pecans, 1/2 apple, 2 cups of water with lemon Crystal Light

LUNCH: turkey breast sandwich, small green salad with a tablespoon of flaxseed oil and lemon, a small peach, iced tea

MID-AFTERNOON MEAL: 1 high-protein bar (32 grams protein), 2 cups of water

DINNER: baked salmon, small baked potato, fresh broccoli, non-fat lemon sorbet, 2 cups of water

Day Two

BREAKFAST: breakfast burrito (made with 4 egg whites, chopped onion, garlic salt and pepper, and a 1/4 of a diced baked potato, and low calorie corn tortillas) Microwave in oven. 1 slice of honey dew melon, green tea, 2 cups of water

MID-MORNING MEAL: 1 glass of protein powder and non-fat milk. A small handful of almonds

"To believe with certainty, we must begin without doubting."–Charles Prosper

LUNCH: tuna salad (made tuna packed in water, with fat-free mayonnaise, dill pickle relish, and fresh lemon juice). Place on a pile of fresh lettuce. A small bunch of grapes. 2 cups of water

MID-AFTERNOON MEAL: 1 high-protein bar (32 grams protein), 2 cups of water

DINNER: baked turkey with 1 tablespoon of cranberry sauce on the side, a portion of brown rice, steamed mixed vegetables, 2 cups of water with peach Crystal Light

Day Three

BREAKFAST: 1 glass of non-fat milk mixed with banana-flavored whey protein powder, fresh strawberries, 1/2 banana, a tablespoon of flaxseed oil, a cup of green tea, 2 cups of water

MID-MORNING MEAL: 1 cup of non-fat cottage cheese, 3 dates, 2 cups of water

LUNCH: breast chicken sandwich, (made with whole wheat bread, fat-free mayo, lettuce and tomatoes, relish) apple, iced tea

DINNER: broiled rainbow trout, steamed spinach, baked potato, scoop of non-fat frozen strawberry sorbet, 2 cups of water with peach Crystal Light

Day Four

BREAKFAST: 1 small bowl of grits, 1 egg omelette (Made with 4 egg whites, low-fat cheddar cheese, chopped bell pepper and onions) 1 persimmon, green tea, 2 cups of water

MID-MORNING MEAL: 1 cup of non-fat milk, cottage cheese and blueberries, a small handful of walnuts, 2 cups of water

LUNCH: 1 veggie burger, steamed green beans, 2 cups of water

MID-AFTERNOON MEAL: 1 high-protein bar (32 grams protein), 2 cups of water

"You'll see it when you believe it."–Wayne Dyer

DINNER: shrimp cocktail with cocktail sauce and lemon, 1 baked potato, raspberry frozen non-fat sorbet, 2 cups of water with stawberry-kiwi flavored Crystal Light

Day Five

BREAKFAST: 1 glass of non-fat milk mixed with banana-flavored whey protein powder, fresh strawberries, 1/2 banana, a tablespoon of flaxseed oil, a cup of green tea, 2 cups of water

MID-MORNING MEAL: 1 glass of non-fat milk mixed with chocolate-flavored whey protein powder, a small handful of almonds

LUNCH: broiled rainbow trout, (served with fat-free mayo and lemon) brown rice, iced tea

MID-AFTERNOON MEAL: 1 high-protein bar (32 grams protein), 2 cups of water

DINNER: grilled halibut, steamed string beans and carrots, 1 yam, frozen non-fat blueberry sorbet, 2 cups of water with cola flavored Crystal Light

Day Six

BREAKFAST: 4 scrambled egg whites (Made with Pam non-stick cooking spray), 1 cup of Cream of Wheat, 1/2 orange, 1 cup of green tea, 2 cups of water

MID-MORNING MEAL: 1 glass of protein powder and non-fat milk. a small handful of walnuts

LUNCH: turkey breast sandwich (made with whole wheat bread, fat-free mayonnaise, dill pickle relish, lettuce and tomatoes), a small plum, 2 cups of water

MID-AFTERNOON MEAL: 1 high-protein bar (32 grams protein), 2 cups of water

DINNER: broiled orange roughy fish, red beans and brown rice, 1 cup of lemon frozen non-fat sorbet, 2 cups of water with tea-flavored Crystal Light

"Solutions depend on how you define the problem."–
Charles Prosper

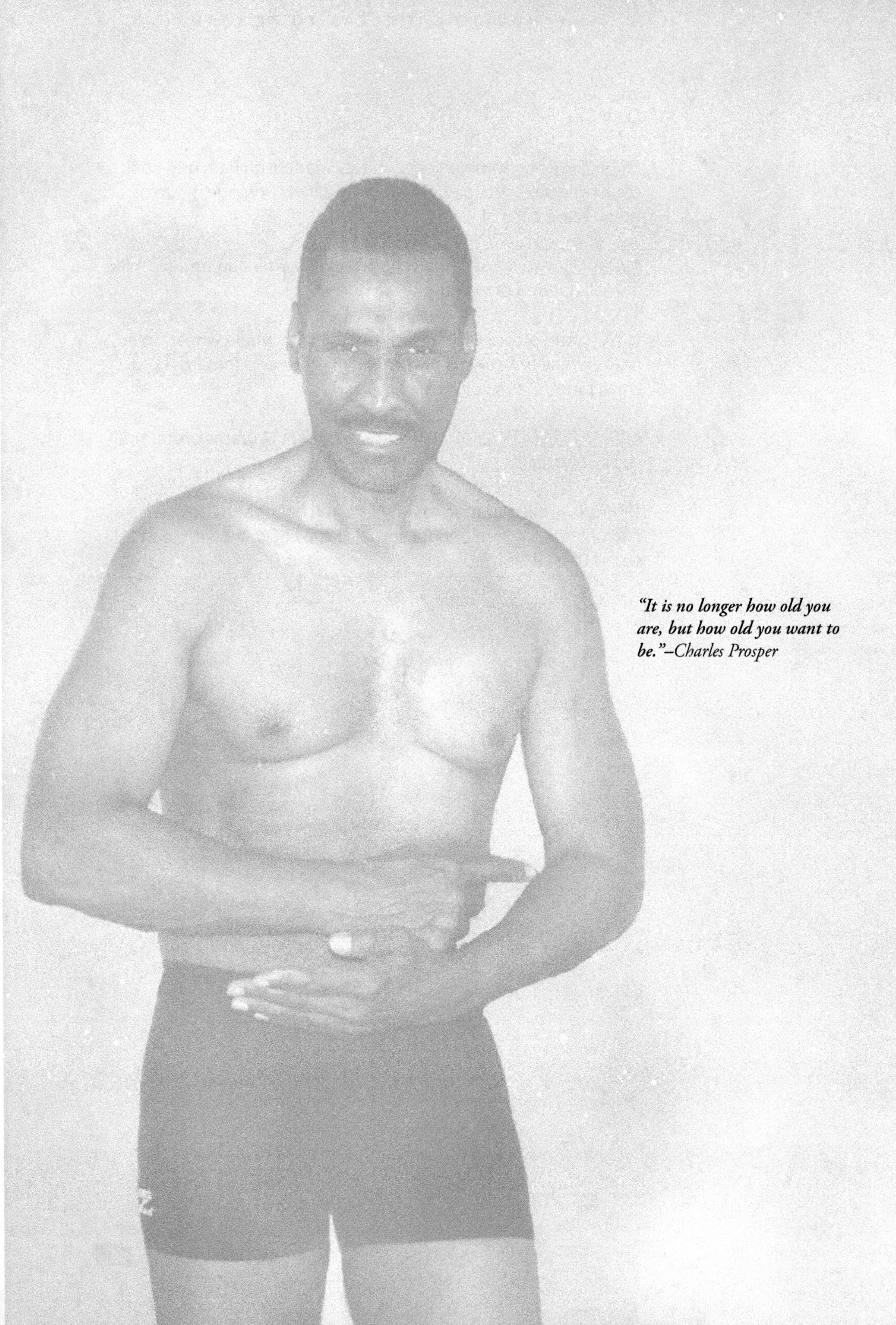

"It is no longer how old you are, but how old you want to be."–Charles Prosper

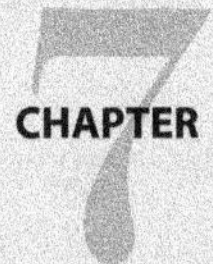

CHAPTER 7

How To Get Fat Fast - Forget All The Fit After Fifty Stuff

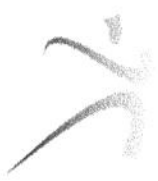

Wait a minute. I realize that there are people out there, that for whatever reason, picked up this book and think that I am full of you-know-what with all of this discipline, discipline, discipline in being lean, fit and all of that. Hey, what if you don't give a hoot about what you eat? What if you want to see how much weight you can put on by eating everything that you want? Okay, I will suppose that you, the reader, in some parallel universe have decided that you want to eat in order to get fat fast. Who knows. Maybe you just landed a movie role playing Santa Claus in a new sci-fi action thriller "Attack of the Reindeer". Well, in this chapter, I will show you exactly how to put on the maximum amount of weight in the shortest amount of time. Let us start with some basic rules, then I will show you where to go and exactly what to eat.

"Success is when you do what you say you're going to do."–Emily Ruth Goins

The Top 5 Rules for Gaining Weight As Fast As Possible

These 5 simple rules will get you to your goal faster than anything you could ever imagine:

- **Rule Number 1** - Don't exercise. Just do only the movements that it takes to pick up one more potato chip after another (with cheese dip of course) while *watching* athletes on TV perform, who of course are in top physical shape. Just watching these superb athletes will suffice.

- **Rule Number 2** - Skip breakfast. However, if you *do* have breakfast, make sure that it is something delightful like a Danish and coffee (with sugar and cream of course).

- **Rule Number 3** - Enjoy the grease. Stay away from all of that trendy low-fat stuff. Real men eat grease.

- **Rule Number 4** - Eat late - then go to sleep. Hey, look, if you've worked hard all day, you deserve a a nice large cheese and sausage pizza to go along with that ice cold bottle of beer. Ahh!

- **Rule Number 5** - Eat Fast Food. Why cook! You must know and use all of your fast food options. But what are your fat-food options? Oops! I meant to say *fast*-food options.

Before we look at the most popular fast food chains and what they serve, let us recall what the get-lean-and-healthy crowd are doing – and just do the opposite.

To be lean, a person must:

- Eat five small meals a day
- Keep each meal at around 500 calories (no more than 600)
- Make sure that the calories from fat are 20% to 25%
- Keep the total day's calories between 2000 to 2500 calories
- Exercise with progressive weight resistance and cardio exercise

"You will always find time for that which you love to do-no matter how 'busy' you are."–Charles Prosper

Well, the exercising part should be no problem because it is a simple matter of *not* doing it! But what are the places that I am most likely to get fattest the fastest? Let's take a stroll through Fast Food Lane. But first, let me show you a little math trick that will allow you to quickly know the percent of the calories from fat by just knowing the **Total Calories** of the meal and the **Fat Grams** contained in the meal.

This is the formula. *Every gram of fat is the same as 9 calories.* Let me repeat that. **Every gram of fat is the same as 9 calories**. What does this mean? This means that we have a simple multiplication problem. Let me give you a problem. Let's say that a certain food has **670 Total Calories**, and it says that it has *40 grams of fat*. Well, if every gram of fat is the same as 9 calories, you would simply multiply:

9 x 40 = **360 Calories from Fat**

Now, to find the % of fat calories which should be only 20% to lose weight, we only need to divide the Total Calories into the Calories from Fat.

360 / 670 = **54%**

54% fat calories is way more than our lean 20% calories from fat!

Eating this meal - with more than half of the calories as fat-calories is a guaranteed dead ringer to get you fat if you consistently eat it on a regular basis. Oh, and by the way, just in case you're a little curious, what I just gave you are the Total Calories and the Calories from Fat of The Original **Whopper** Hamburger from **Burger King**®. But wait! There' more.

McDonald's® (A Typical Meal)

	Cals	Fat grams	Fat Cals	% Fat Cals
Big Mac	540	29	261	48%
Large Fries	500	25	225	45%
Med. Coke®	210	0	0	0%
	1260			

"The best way to escape from any problem is to solve it."–Anonymous

Are you able to see what I see? To be lean, one needs the % Fat Cals to be at around 20%. With the case of having a Big Mac and Large Fries we are way over 20% – at 48% and 45%. It is supposed that each meal should be around 500 to 600 calories at any one sitting because this is about the maximum number of calories that the body can process and use at any one meal. Anything over 500 or 600 calories gets stored away as fat. That is you get to wear those 760 calories around your waist. If you forgot how we get the Fat Cals (Fat Calories), remember that every gram of fat is equivalent to 9 calories, so I simply multiplied 29 x 9 = 261 and 25 x 9 = 225. Then it was just a matter of dividing respectively 261 by 540 and dividing 225 by 500 to get 48% and 45%. Having, say three meals like this one in a day, would spell about 3780 Total Daily Calories. This is far above the recommended 2000 to 2500 Daily Calorie recommended intake. So, at 3780 calories per day, it would be *very* easy to super-size yourself.

Now before I expound on KFC®, can anybody tell me why they don't want to say the "F"–word any more? You know what I'm talking about. They used to say Kentucky *Fried* Chicken®. What's with the shameful abbreviations? If I say "F-you", you still know what I mean. Anyway, I digress. Let us look at a meal from, *ahem!* - KFC®.

KFC® (Extra Crispy Meal)

	Cals	Fat grams	Fat Cals	% Fat Cals
Breast	490	31	279	57%
Thigh	370	27	243	66%
Potato Wedges	260	13	117	45%
Biscuit	180	8	72	40%
	1300			

After breakfast, if you have really got a man-sized appetite (or a big-woman-sized appetite, you first stop should be to the nearest Del Taco®. Here, I am sure that we can put together a calorie-rich, fat feast of a meal in no time flat. Hmmm. Let's see. How about? –

Del Taco® (Macho Beef Burrito)

	Cals	Fat grams	Fat Cals	% Fat Cals
Burrito	1010	44	396	39%
Small Fries	270	16	144	53%
Choc. Shake	600	13	117	20%
	1880			

Let's do our analysis of this meal. The lean goal is to have the total calories of the meal from 500 to 600 calories. At 1880 calories, we have achieved *more than double* the recommended portion. The total amount of calories for the entire day should be between 2000 and 2500 calories. A days worth of calories is happening with just this one meal. What is our limit for % Fat Cals to be lean? 20% right? Well, over limits at 39% Fat Cals and 53% Fat Cals. But wait. What do I see? Only 20% Fat Cals for the Chocolate Shake. But "Holy Smokes!", there are 600 calories in that shake - equivalent to a full meal in itself. Remember the rule: Low Fat + High Calories = Gain Weight Fast.

"It is not how much you have but how much you enjoy that creates happiness." *–Anonymous*

I used to eat breakfast at Denny's® almost everyday, and I had a waist to prove it. To pop some pants buttons sooner than you think, try this for breakfast

Denny's® (Breakfast)

	Cals	Fat grams	Fat Cals	% Fat Cals
Two Eggs Over	200	15	135	67%
Hashed Browns	200	12	108	54%
Bacon (3 slices)	125	10	90	72%
English Muffin	133	1.5	13.5	10%
Orange Juice	110	0.5	4.5	3%
	768			

Pop question. Is there anything on this menu that you could eat that would not get you fat? If you just had the English Muffin and the orange juice you'd be fine, calorie and fat-wise. However, if you added scrambled egg whites, you'd have put together for yourself an à la carte, lean and clean meal, *assuming of course that losing weight were important to you.*

Okay, maybe I have been giving examples that are a little extreme in the way of an appetite. Let's try just 3 slices of pepperoni pizza and a medium cola. I think that's reasonable to look at as a typical American meal.

Pizza Hut® (3 slices of pepperoni pizza)

	Cals	Fat grams	Fat Cals	% Fat Cals
1 slice p. pizza	200	9	81	41%
1 slice p. pizza	200	9	81	41%
1 slice p. pizza	200	9	81	41%
1 med. cola	210	0	0	0%
	810			

Well, even three slices of pizza and a soda will put us over the limit again. We are over 210 calories of what should be eaten for one meal, and the % Fat Cals is way over the healthy norm of 20% – for a slice of pepperoni pizza, it is a whopping 41%.

"To know which direction to take next, you must first accept where you now are."–Anonymous

Hey, I am from the south where Southern fried chicken rules – (so I have the incidents of heart attacks and strokes in my family: my first aunt died of a stroke as well as my mother.) *Anyway,* if we are going to do Southern fried chicken, we have to do Southern fried chicken *right* by visiting Popeye's® Chicken.

Popeye's®

	Cals	Fat grams	Fat Cals	% Fat Cals
Chciken Breast	355	21	189	53%
Chicken Wing	145	10	90	62%
Red Beans/Rice	320	19	171	53%
Apple Turnover	250	12	108	43%
1 med. cola	210	0	0	0%
	1280			

Bring out the Spandex and unbutton your belt. You belly is going to have a party tonight! Everything, including the cola, will turn you from hard-body to lard-body. Even though the cola has no fat calories – it does have a *lot* of refined sugar – for a 12 oz. Coca Cola or Pepsi – you get to ingest 10 teaspoons of sugar. Just for the fun of it – try to imagine yourself swallowing 10 teaspoons of sugar straight from the bag. Just the thought of this should give you the jitters. Simple sugars found in colas quickly convert to fat cells in the body. Sugar = Fat.

Maybe the high fat in fast food is typical of only American locations. Let's do Japanese for a change, and see what happens. I know. Let's go to Yoshinoya®. I hear their beef bowl is terrific.

Yoshinoya®

	Cals	Fat grams	Fat Cals	% Fat Cals
1 Beef Bowl®	685	27	243	36%
1 clam chowder	210	9	81	38%
1 med. cola	210	0	0	0%
	1105			

36% Fat Calories and 38% Fat Calories is still too high over the lean target norm of 20 to 25%. And look at those Total Calories for this meal – 1105 calories. Now I know where Sumo wrestlers go to get their girth.

Dodo Bird Alert!

Though I should not have to say this, but this entire chapter was meant as a satire – a joke! If taken literally as advice on how to eat will probably put you in the hospital or the grave if you indulge yourself like this on a daily or regular basis. I repeat. I wrote it only and all in fun!

"We don't see things as they are, we see them as we are."–Anaïs Nin

WARNING: Do NOT try to eat these foods at home alone – or without a doctor's supervision.

I feel I need to take this warning up a notch with a formal disclamer. Here goes:

IMPORTANT DISCLAIMER

- The publisher and author of this book are not medical doctors capable and licensed to give you medical advice. You should always consult your medical professional for medical advice before making any type of medical or health decision based on any information that you may read in this book.

- This book was researched and compiled for educational purposes only for other sources believed to be accurate and reliable. Food manufacturers are constantly changing their products, this information, though believed accurate at the time of this writing, is subject to change as the food manufacturers change their products. The food manufacturers, in the end, are the final authorities on the food's most up to date nutrition facts information.

- If you are matching your insulin dosage to carbohydrate intake, you should not rely on the figures given in this book. You should always check the food labels and/or contact the food manufacturer for the most current nutritional information for your own safety.

- The information that is provided here in this book is provided "As Is" and does not have any warranty expressed or implied. The author and publisher expressly disclaim any liability that may or could arise from the use or misuse of the information in this book. All consequential, special, incidental, indirect, direct, or punitive damages that may or could arise from the use or misuse of the information in this book is excluded and disclaimed.

"I do not want to be happy. I want to be at peace, for only once I am at peace can I truly be happy."–*Charles Prosper*

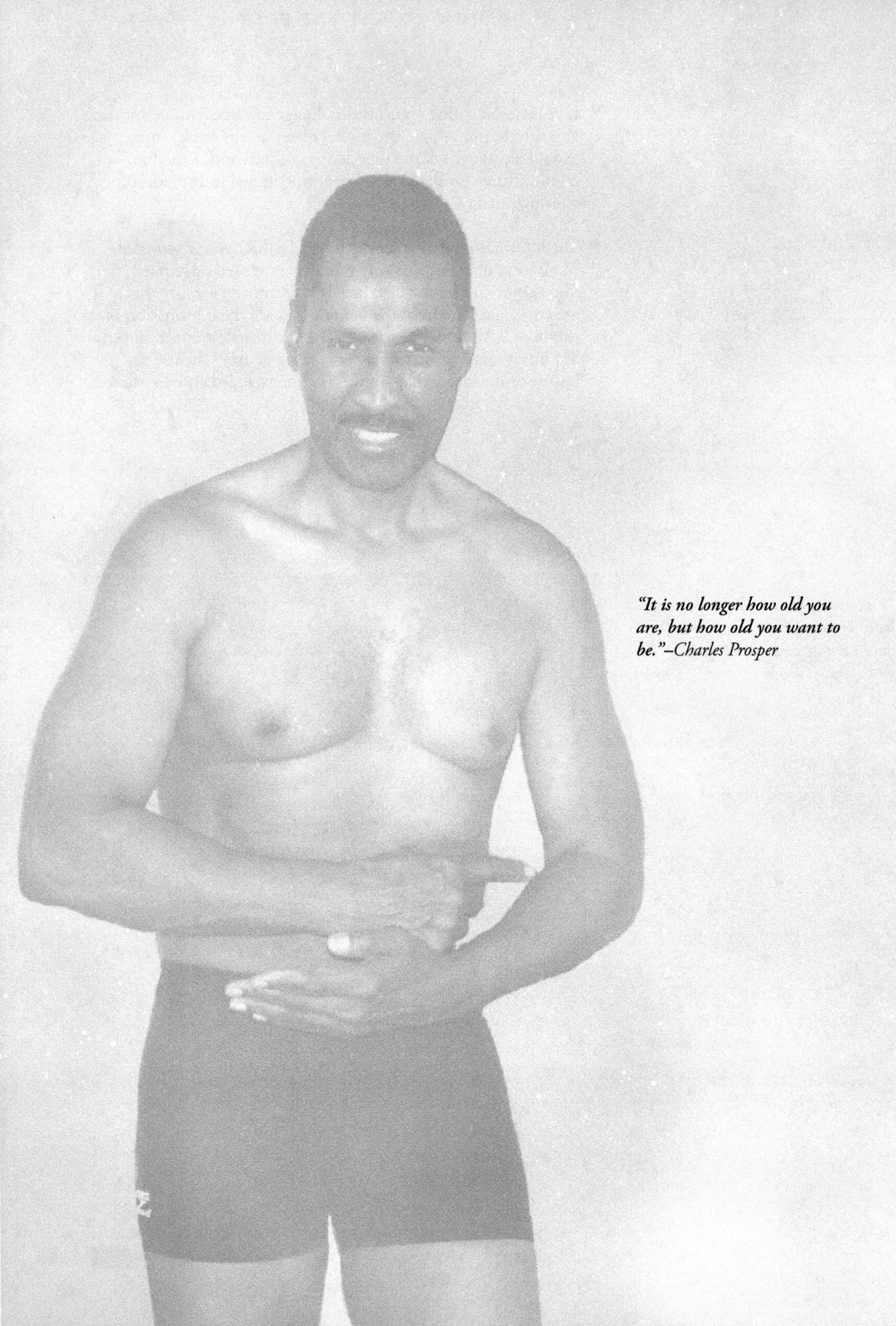

"It is no longer how old you are, but how old you want to be."–Charles Prosper

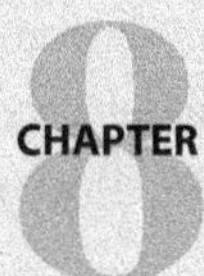
CHAPTER 8

Frequently Asked Questions (FAQ)

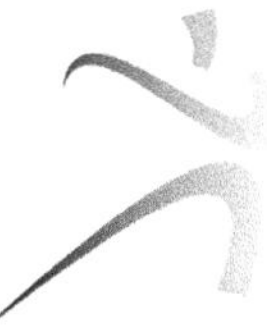

In this chapter, I would like to address and answer some of the popular queries and confusions surrounding health, fitness and longevity. My aim is to make the seemingly complicated as simple and as understandable as possible. So, let's get right down to it with one of my favorites – the question of antioxidants and "free radicals".

"Life affords no higher pleasure than that of surmounting difficulties."–Samuel Johnson

Q: What are antioxidants? Really. And what the heck are free radicals? These terms sound cool to say, but nobody appears to give me a good answer when I ask exactly what does this mean?

C.P. The word antioxidant as well as the word free radicals are thrown around a lot with the majority of people who use them, generally speaking, don't have *a clue* what they are talking about. Think I'm kidding? Just go to any health or nutrition store, and ask the clerk or whoever claims to be the in-store resident guru and ask them: "What is an anti-oxidant?" I will guarantee that the first thing that they say is something like: "Oh, sure. You need them to fight the free radicals in your body." Well, excuse me! Now you have introduced two words, neither of which have been adequately defined or explained.

To understand what is an anti-oxidant or a free radical, you must have an understanding of basic high school chemistry at the molecular level.

Anti-oxidant theory is based on the way a healthy oxygen molecule is supposed to behave within your body at the cellular molecular level. Let's review your high school chemistry. An atom is the smallest theoretical particle of matter. An atom is comprised of a nucleus of particles called *protons*, and revolving around the nucleus, like planets circling the sun, we have the particles called *electrons*. Now here is the key. There must be an equality in number of the protons with the electrons, that is to say, if there are 8 protons, for a healthy normal atom, there must be revolving around these 8 protons also 8 corresponding electrons. The number of the neutrons must equal the number of electrons. Two (or more) atoms joined together becomes a *molecule*. In the case of oxygen, join two oxygen atoms – and you get – *ta da!* – an *oxygen molecule*. This is a healthy oxygen molecule. Due to toxins and pollutants that we breathe in the air, these enviromental poisons cause electrons to destabilize, that is, to break off a normal oxygen molecule, and thus causing it to be *short* an electron. Now, this molecule has become deranged and unstable. Because it does not have an even number and balance of electrons to match with the number of protons, it becomes – the piranha of oxygen molecules which we call a – *free radical*. Now these free radical molecules are searching for an extra electron that they can "steal" from other cell tissue. This consequently causes a domino effect from every molecule that gets its electron stolen, in turn, becomes a "free radical" molecule also (kind like when a werewolf bites you, you become a werewolf also). This domino effect can wreck havoc to healthy tissue within the body resulting in premature aging, destruction of DNA and even clogging of the arteries. Who can save us? Antioxidants to the rescue! Antioxidants which are found in fresh foods like vegetables and fruits, in supplements which contain vitamin A, C , E and beta carotene, act like a giant wall or boulder standing in front of the path of free radicals, stopping their damaging activity. If you would like to see a visual representation of this explanation, see below and the next page.

"You are the one who must choose your place."–James Lane Allen

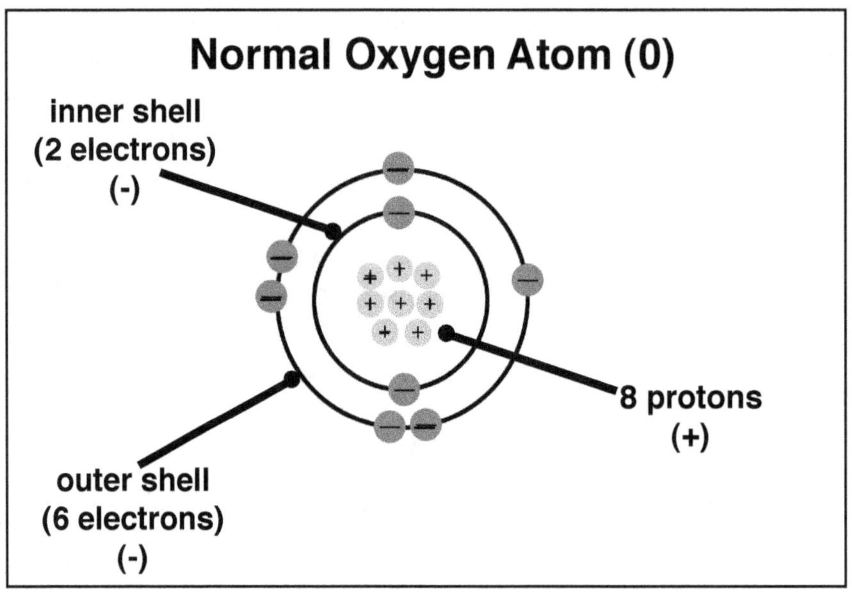

(protons = electrons)

Normal Oxygen Molecule (0^2)

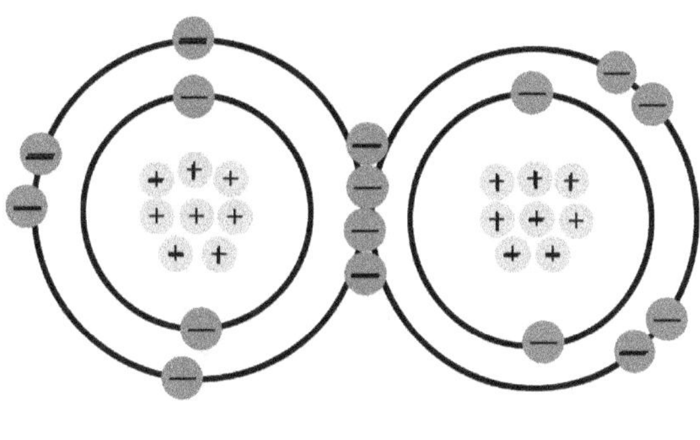

0 = 0

filled outer shell
(inert)

"That old law about "an eye for an eye" leaves everybody blind."–Martin Luther King, Jr.

What you see here is a normal *(inert)* molecule that is joined together by two normal oxygen *atoms*. (Remember, two or more atoms joined together makes a *molecule* – the next-level unit-up.)

Free Radical Oxygen Molecule (0^2)

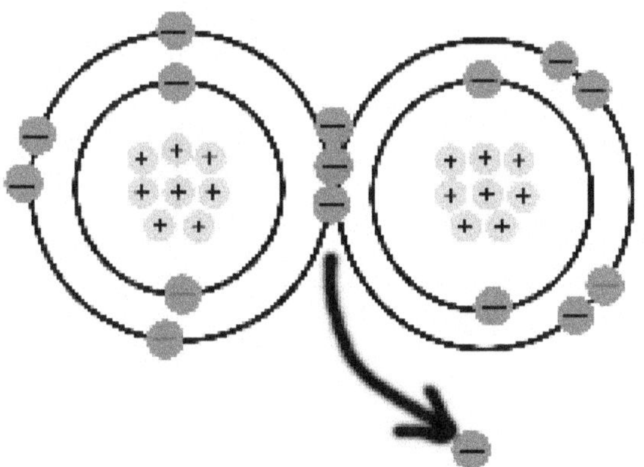

Here we can see how a normal oxygen molecule has become a damaged molecule by losing one of its electrons. Ladies and gentlemen, this molecule, which is now missing an electron which has broken off, has now become a ravaging, roaming *free radical.*

Q: Charles, I am a woman of 51. I like the idea of getting lean and firm, but I don't want to life weights and look muscular like a man.

C.P. The only way that you could ever obtain the extreme musculature of a professional female bodybuilder is if you take male steroids which, though reticent to admit, they most certainly do. You will get toned, firmed and curvy when you add progressive weight resistance to your regimen. Firm shapely muscle on a female body is oh so sexy!

Q: Will I have to go on a diet in order to lose weight and be successful with your Fit Fast System?

C.P. My ears! My ears! You're hurting my ears! You said *diet!* No, we don't do the D-word with my system. You don't eat less – you eat *more* – as many as 5 small meals a day. This way you are *never* hungry, and you are never sacrificing. Diets are temporary paths to guaranteed failure. With my system, you only change the way you eat which has nothing at all to do with *being on a diet.*

"The true object of all human life is play."–G.K. Chesterton

Q: How long will it take for me to see results?

C.P. If you follow to the T everything as planned and clearly laid out for you – you will see a *dramatic* change in as little as *12 weeks!*

Q: How often will I have to exercise?

C.P. You will work out with your weights, your barbells and dumbbells for two consecutive days followed by a day of cardio or aerobic exercise. You will be doing *some* sort of exercise everyday.

Q: How long will I have to spend in the gym each workout?

C.P. You can develop a fabulous body working out for only 45 minutes each workout. On your jogging or aerobics day, you need only spend 20 to 30 minutes.

Q: How strict do I have to be with my new eating habits?

C.P. You will learn how to eat clean and healthy, 5 times a day for 6 days a week – then guess what happens on the 7th day? On the 7th day, or whatever the one day of the week that you select – you eat what ever you want. If you want some french fries on that day – go for it. A piece of pie? Fine. This is called eating your "cheat meal" on your cheat day.

Q: Do I need to enroll in a gym, or can I just purchase some barbells and dumbbells and workout at home?

C.P. You most definitely can create your own home gym if you like. Though I have belonged to professional gyms, for the last 3 years, I personally have worked out in my garden, outside in the open air, and have made tremendous gains and progress while loving the beauty and solitude of it every moment. It's a personal call. Either will do.

Q: I haven't worked out in years, and I am 63, is it safe for me to begin to exercise?

C.P. No matter what physical condition you are in, and no matter if you are over 40, you should always get a preliminary check up with your doctor first, and once he gives you the okay, you should be fine.

Q: I am a man now in his sixties, will your system improve my sex drive?

C.P. If you follow faithfully my system, progressive weight resistance along with proper eating and rest *will* put lead in your pencil – at 60, 70 or 80.

"Nothing can bring you peace but yourself."–Ralph Waldo Emerson

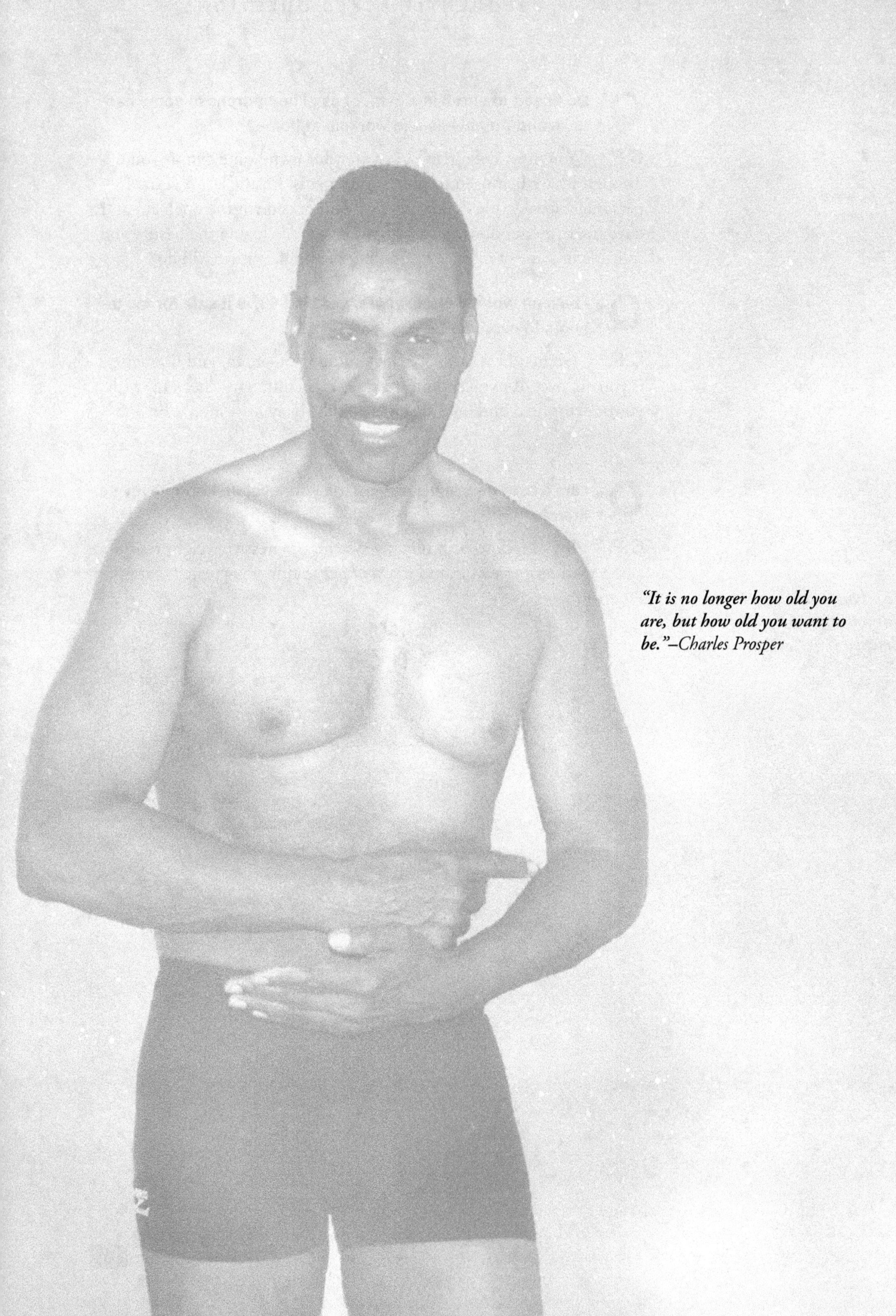

"It is no longer how old you are, but how old you want to be."–Charles Prosper

The Importance of Goal-Setting

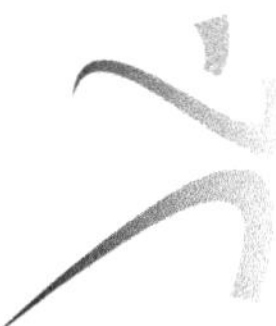

And what about goals? Are they important to the achieving of my ideal body? Absolutely yes! Establishing a goal, making a plan and following through on that plan is probably as important if not more so than the actual plan itself. You see, a system, a method or a plan is just a tool to get you from here to there by removing or solving a problem. A hammer doesn't hammer - *you* hammer with the hammer. All tools - as is knowledge - are inert and powerless until - *you* - the ultimate doer take action on it. What makes anyone take action on anything and then stick to it until its completion? Three things: desire, a goal and a plan of action. Desire is the fuel. The goal is the why. And the plan of action is the how. In this chapter I want to talk about the why, that is, I want to talk about the importance of your setting and staying with your goal until completion.

"The only way to get rid of a problem is to solve it."–Dale Haynesworth

Why You Must Have Goals

A man without a goal is like a ship without a rudder. I think you would agree that if you got inside of a motor boat with no guiding rudder in a harbor, rev it up and let it go wheresoever, once it took off into the open waters the chances of crashing into the rocks, capsizing or smashing into another boat would be the very likely fate of such a foolish dis-embarkment. But isn't this exactly what we do with our lives when we go along day-by-day hoping that something better will happen to us or at least nothing worse in life will befall us? This is called living by default. Living by default assumes that there is nothing that you *can* do to make your life better. And if you *know* what you can do and don't do it, your life is no better than a person who doesn't know.

Goals work as does the magnifying glass. Place a piece of paper on the sidewalk in the bright sun on a clear summer day. Stand there for about an hour or two and see what happens. Assuming that you secured the paper to the ground with a weight on the edge of it, it will still be there, little warmer perhaps, but unchanged. Now take out a magnifying glass and point it onto the center of the paper and pull the magnifying glass back, a little, and just a little more until the light spot that is beamed onto the paper begins to sizzle, within seconds, and thus burns a hole through it. The magnifying glass takes the rays of the sun and concentrates it onto the paper, such that now those same warm sun rays can do things that it could not until it was concentrated. Thus is the power of goals. Goals are the magnifying glass which take the infinite powers of your mind and concentrate them with such power that they can burn and cut through any obstacle set before it. There is nothing more powerful than a made up mind with a goal at the forefront.

I first heard the following example by the great motivational speaker, Zig Ziglar, and I want to give you my synopsis of it. Let us take the world's greatest archer, someone who, say, could hit a bull's-eye 10 out of 10 times from a hundred yards away with a bow and arrow. I can show you a way to out-shoot this professional archer even though you have never picked up a bow and arrow. How? Easy. Just blindfold this archer, spin him around a few times, and ask him to shoot. Sounds silly doesn't it? You are surely asking yourself right now. "How can he hit a target he can't even see?" Well, I have an even better question for you. "How can ***you*** hit a target that you don't even have?" You must have your goals.

"Forgiveness is the fragrance that the violet leaves on the heel that crushes it."–Mark Twain

Now there is another trap that you can fall into. Some people confuse activity with accomplishment. Some load up there lives with all sorts of insignificant time wasting activities that they literally crowd out the days of their lives making it impossible to achieve anything significant. You must first know and define what is important to you. Then you must start about with plans and steps to its accomplishment. (More on this a little later in this chapter.) Do you know what a processional caterpillar is? It is a furry little caterpillar which follows unquestionably the caterpillar in front of it. The assumption is that the first caterpillar in the line (and sometimes there may be dozens of caterpillars following each other) knows where the food is or is at least the one on alert and looking for it. A scientist tried an experiment. He found a row of processional caterpillars traveling along a wood trail. He directed the first caterpillar to follow the back of the last caterpillar until all of the caterpillars formed a perfect circle, following each other round and round and round. He put some pine needles, food for caterpillars, in the middle of the circle. The caterpillars followed each other in circles for hours, days, until they all literally dropped dead from exhaustion when the goal, the food, the pine needles was right in their midst. When you do not set your own agenda, that is, set and follow your own goal, you become swept away by the agenda and thinking of the masses. Without a goal, you become just like the processional caterpillar, doing what others do, going where others go and having what others have.

What Is Your Health and Fitness Goal?

Whatever your answer is, I want you to do something very important.

I want you to take out a small plain index card, and I want you to *write* down in one clear sentence: your goal, what you plan to do to achieve this goal and when you expect to have achieved this. Here is an example.

My Health and Fitness Goal

I weigh__lbs., By JUne 30, 20__ . I am fit, muscular, toned and strong. I achieve this by regular weight resistance exercises, combined with cardio exercises and clean healthy eating.

X____________________

(Your signature and today's date)

"Faith sees the invisible believes the incredible and receives the impossible." – *Anonymous*

Now, here's your assignment. Every morning and every night for the next 90 days, that is, the next 12 weeks, I want you to read out loud – just once – the above goal commitment. You only need to read it out loud *just once.* I can only say that you will be amazed how this simple exercise of goal-focusing will keep you on track. It will only take you about 20 seconds to read it each time. Small investment for amazing results.

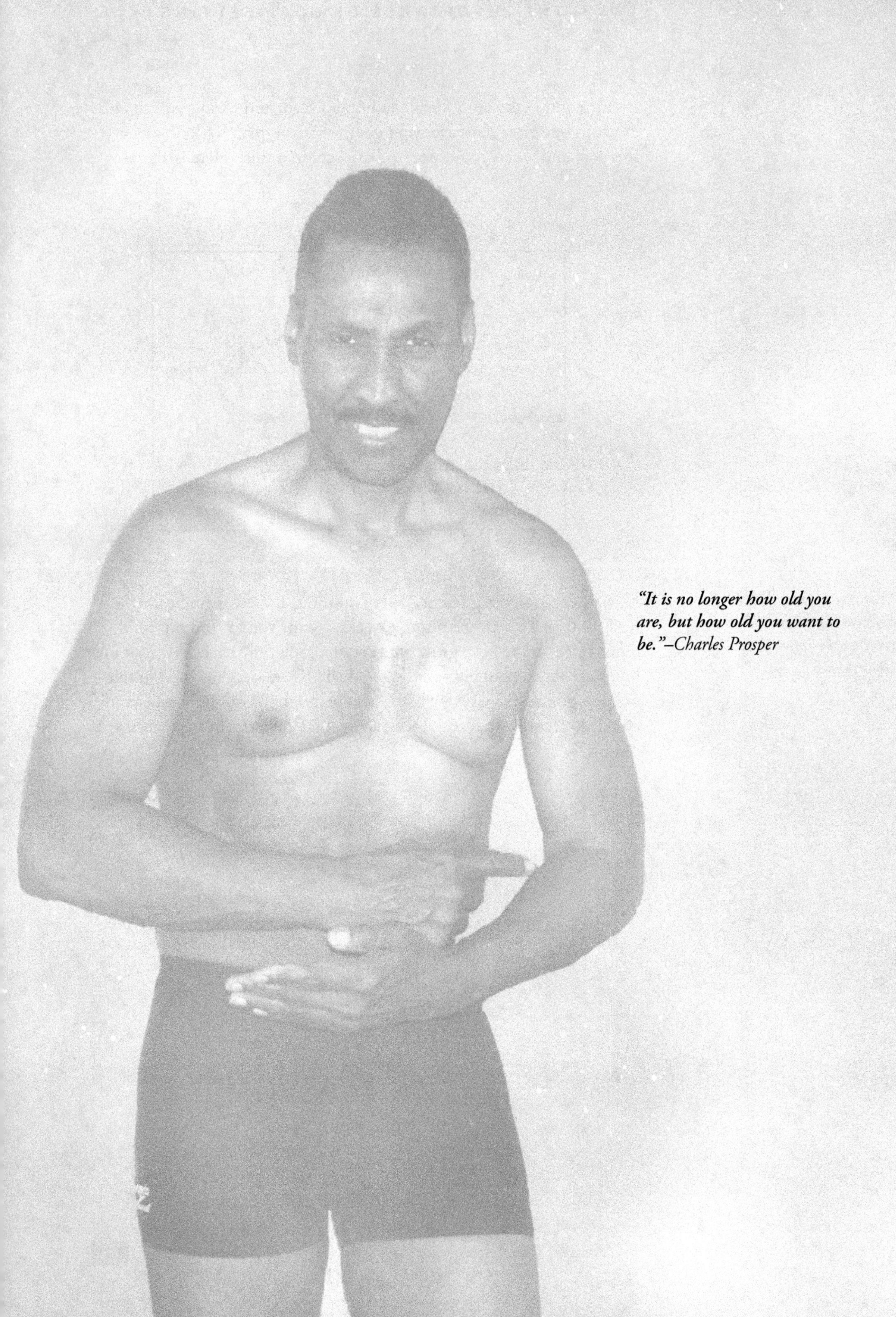

"It is no longer how old you are, but how old you want to be."–Charles Prosper

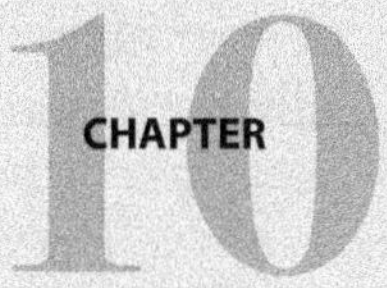

CHAPTER 10

Weight Training Exercises For Fitness Success

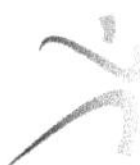

The Prosper Fit Fast System is a 12-week program of change to convince you that this is to be your permanent life style of healthy living. In 12 weeks, if you stick with it, you will be *more than* pleasantly surprised. In this chapter, in addition to many proven and effective weight resistance exercises to choose for each major muscle group, I will also give you an easy to follow *Daily and Monthly Workout Planner* which you can photocopy and place within a carry around 3-ring spiral notebook when you workout and for your future workout planning.

"If you worry about what might be, and wonder what might have been, you will ignore what is."–Anonymous

You Will Do Something Everyday

With the *Prosper Fit Fast System*, you will either be doing, on any given day, weight training or cardio/aerobic exercises. You will soon get used to and even look forward to getting up everyday to exercise. You will understand the first time you truly feel the "endorphin rush" of pleasurable body chemicals rewarding you for what you are doing for your body. Your weight resistance exercises should take no longer than 45 minutes to complete. Your cardio should take no longer than 30 minutes (with a just minimum of 20 minutes).

The 3-Day Cycle of Exercising

This is what your three-day cycle of exercise will look like:

- **Day 1 (A) :** *Weight Resistance Training*
- **Day 2 (B) :** *More Weight Resistance Training*
- **Day 3 (C) :** *Cardio/Aerobic Exercise*

You simply keep repeating this cycle. If and whenever you may have to take a day off, just resume exactly where you left off in the cycle. That is to say that if you had to skip on a (B) workout routine, then tomorrow, you just start the cycle at the (B) workout routine, and continue from there in the (A), (B), (C) pattern – more on this in the following section.

The ABC Workout System

The ABC concept of training is based on the idea of working out *push muscles* on one day, *pull muscles* on another and finally the *kick and crunch muscles* on the third day.

Workout A:

With this group of exercises, you will be working the *push muscles,* that is the muscles that will push your weights *away* from your body. These are the exercises that involve the muscles of the chest, shoulders and the triceps.

Workout B:

Here you will work and develop the *pull muscles.* These are the muscles which pull the weights toward your body, those exercises involving the biceps and the back muscles.

Workout C:

Then finally, we exercise on the third module, your *kick and crunch muscles.* These are the muscles involving the legs, calves and the abdominals.

"Feeling is believing."–Anonymous

Here is how your workout cycle would look as an outline:

Day 1 - Workout A (Monday)
Day 2 - Workout B (Tuesday)
Day 3 - *Aerobics* (Wednesday)

Day 4 - Workout C (Thursday)
Day 5 - Workout A (Friday)
Day 6 - *Aerobics* (Saturday)

Day 7 - Workout B (Sunday)
Day 8 - Workout C (Monday)
Day 9 - *Aerobics* (Tuesday)

If you, say, work out your shoulders and chest on a Monday, then you will be able to allow them *four days* to rest and recuperate, since you will not have to work them out again until Friday. The cardio/aerobic exercise that you have on Wednesday will help to deliver more nutrients to your shoulders and chest muscles and as well flush out all of the nasty toxins that have been stored up in the muscles.

To get a visual of your major muscle groups, please see next page.

"Man makes holy what he believes, as he makes beautiful what he loves."–Ernest Renan

Major Muscle Groups

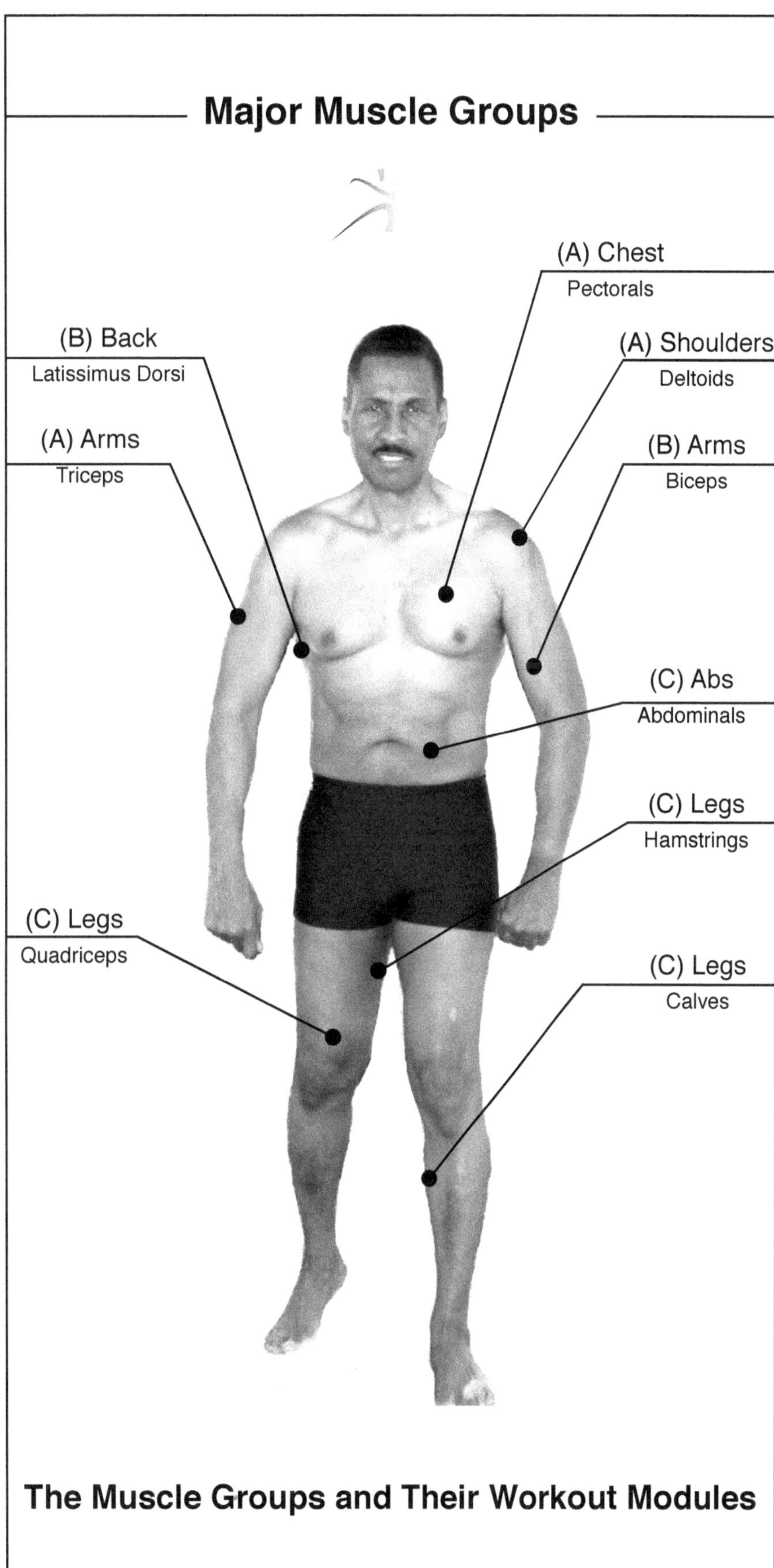

The Muscle Groups and Their Workout Modules

How To Perform Your Exercise Routine

Again, first and foremost, check with your doctor before starting any serious exercise and weight training routine. Once the doc says it's okay, you're ready to start.

The Parlance of Body Building

If you are new to all of this, let me give you some of the lingo and the basics.

A Repetition: A repetition, also known as "reps" is essentially the number of the movements of the exercise whether it is a push, pull, jump or lunge. The number of times you do the movement are called the "reps". If you curl a barbell 10 times, you have done 10 reps.

A Set: The completion of a given number of reps is called a "set". With the *Prosper Fit Fast System*, you will begin by doing 4 sets per exercise, and rest about a minute between each set, or until you catch your breath. The reps for each set of an exercise will vary.

"Some things have to be believed to be seen."–Ralph Hodgson

- The *first set* is a weight that you can comfortably lift for barely 12 reps.
- The *second set,* you use a weight slightly heavier by a few pounds (a little experimentation will let you know), and with this set you will be able to do 10 reps.
- The *third set,* you raise the poundage just a little more, and now you attempt to do 8 reps. (Each workout, you are trying to add as much weight as your new emerging strength will allow.)
- By the *fourth set*, your muscles should be getting tired, and with this last set, you add enough weight that will allow you to barely do 6 reps – but here is where you get intense – *try* to do 7 or 8 reps if you can. With the last set, we exercise with what we call *exercising to failure.* This means that you keep pumping until you just can't do another. Working out with this type of intensity will surely force those muscles to grow. **A Quick Tip:** *Be careful about working your leg muscles to failure.* If you are doing squats, you wouldn't want them to give out on you.

You Must Warm Up By Stretching Before You Begin To Lift

The temptation, when you really get into exercising your body and enjoying the feel of the blood rushing to your muscles, is not to warm up properly for 10 minutes before you start. Look, if you are over 40, or 50, you have to take it easy when you are starting your exercise routine. When your muscles are cold, and you begin full force, is exactly about the time when injuries start to happen. Be safe before you begin by warming up. Later on in the book, I will show you some great stretching and warm up exercises. You will find these in the section on weight resistance exercises. These preliminary stretching exercises will keep your muscles strong, supple and elastic.

The Rev-Up Program

"But wait," you say to me. "Charles, I haven't done any serious exercise for years. I am in terrible shape to just outright and start." No worries. I got your back. What I want you to do is a light workout that will allow you to *ease* your way into some intense training later on. You might call this "training to train". I want to get you ready by having you do a "Rev-Up Program". Before you start your "full-all out" 12-Week Program, you will do "The Rev-Up Program" for only 2 weeks. (I have the complete descriptions of these exercises later on in the section of this chapter where I explain in detail the movements of each.)

"Look well into thyself; there is a source which will always spring up if thou wilt search there."–Marcus Aurelius

All you need to do is to perform 10 to 12 reps of each exercise. Pause for a moment - only long enough to catch your breath - then quickly go to the next one and the next one doing 10 to 12 reps each for each exercise until you finish:

1. Bent-Over Barbell Row (Back)
2. Standing Barbell Curls (Biceps)
3. Abdominal Crunches (Abs)
4. Bench Press (Chest)
5. Seated Dumbell Press (Shoulders)
6. Lying Dumbell Triceps Extension (Triceps)
7. Leg Extensions (Legs - Front Thigh)
8. Leg Curls (Legs - Hamstrings)
9. Standing Dumbbell Calf Raises (Calves)

The next day you do 20 minutes of cardio, jogging or stationary bicycle. The following day, you go back to doing your Rev-Up Routine. Then cardio again. Then next day after cardio, do the Rev-Up Routine again. Keep this pattern of one day Rev-Up – Next Day Cardio for two weeks. After the 2 weeks, you will be ready for the full course.

On the following pages are your Progress Planners. The blank ones are for you to copy.

Fit Fast Exercise Planner

	Group 1	Group 2
Workout A chest	• dumbbell bench press • bench press • inclined dumbbell bench press	• flat bench flyes • inclined dumbbell bench flyes
Workout A shoulders	• standing barbell press • seated dumbbell press • seated barbell press	• bent-over seated side laterals • standing dumbell side laterals
Workout A arms (triceps)	• lying dumbbell triceps extensions • lying barbell triceps extensions	• triceps floor push-ups • bench dips
Workout B back	• one-arm dumbbell rows • wide-grip door chin ups • barbell deadlifts	• bent-over dumbbell rows • bent-over barbell rows
Workout B arms (biceps)	• standing dumbbell curls • standing barbell curls	• seated alternate dumbbell curls • standing alternate dumbbell curls • alternate dumbbell hammer curls
Workout B arms (forearms)	• barbell wrist curls • dumbell wrist curls	• barbell reverse wrist curls • dumbell reverse wrist curls • barbell standing reverse curls
Workout C legs (quadriceps)	• barbell squats • dumbbell squats	• leg extensions (bench attachment) • dumbbell lunges
Workout C legs (hamstrings)	• leg curls (bench attachment) • dumbbell lunges	• straight-leg barbell deadlifts • straight-leg dumbbell deadlifts
Workout C legs (calves)	• two-dumbbell calf-raises • seated barbell toe raises	• barbell standing calf-raises • one-legged dumbbell calf-raises
Workout C abdominals	• declined sit-ups • adominal floor crunches	• lying bench leg raises • hanging leg raises

The compendium of possible exercises goes far beyond this list, but it's a start. Simply look for the body part you want to exercise, and select one execise from the first group and another exercise from the second group. Then go for it!

Monthly Workout Progress Planner

Month: January

1	2	3	4	5	6	7
	A	B	X	C	A	X
8	9	10	11	12	13	14
B	C	O	A	B	X	C
15	16	17	18	19	20	21
A	X	B	C	X	A	B
22	23	24	25	26	27	28
X	C	A	X	B	C	X
29	30	31				
A	B	X				

A: Chest, Shoulders, Triceps
B: Back, Biceps, Forearms
C: Legs, Abs
X: Cardio/Aerobics
O: Off Day

NOTES

- **You do two consecutive days** of weight training, that is, (A, B, or C). Two consecutive days of training is then followed by one day of Cardio/Aerobics (X). You simply repeat this cycle of two days weight training rotating with one day of aerobics. If you happen to take an Off Day (O), just continue the next workout where you last left off.

Monthly Workout Progress Planner

Month: ________________

1	2	3	4	5	6	7
8	9	10	11	12	13	14
15	16	17	18	19	20	21
22	23	24	25	26	27	28
29	30	31				

A: Chest, Shoulders, Triceps
B: Back, Biceps, Forearms
C: Legs, Abs
X: Cardio/Aerobics
O: Off Day

NOTES

- **You do two consecutive days** of weight training, that is, (A, B, or C). Two consecutive days of training is then followed by one day of Cardio/Aerobics (X). You simply repeat this cycle of two days weight training rotating with one day of aerobics. If you happen to take an Off Day (O), just continue the next workout where you last left off.

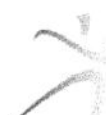

Workout C: Legs • Calves • Abs

Daily Workout Progress Planner

Date: 12/4/09	Planned Start Time: 5:00 a.m.	Actual Start Time: 5:10 a.m.
Day: Thursday	Planned End Time: 5:45 a.m.	Actual End Time: 5:57 a.m.
Legs • Calves • Abs	Estimated to Complete: 42 minutes	Total Time Taken: 47 minutes

Workout C	Exercise	PLAN Reps	PLAN Weight (lbs.)	PLAN Minutes Between Sets	ACTUAL Reps	ACTUAL Weight (lbs.)	NOTES
Legs	Seated Leg Extensions	12	70	1	12	70 −	
	Seated Leg Extensions	10	80	1	10	80 −	
	Seated Leg Extensions	8	90	1	8	90 −	
	Seated Leg Extensions	6	100	2	6	100 −	Less 5 lbs.
Legs	Lying Leg Curls	12	45	1	12	45 +	
	Lying Leg Curls	10	55	1	10	55 +	
	Lying Leg Curls	8	65	1	8	65 +	
	Lying Leg Curls	6	75	2	6	75 +	Add 5 lbs.
Calves	Standing Barbell Calf Raises	12	110	1	12	110	
	Standing Barbell Calf Raises	10	120	1	10	120	
	Standing Barbell Calf Raises	8	130	1	8	130	
	Standing Barbell Calf Raises	6	140	2	6	140	
Calves	One-Leg Dumbell Raise	12	30	1	12	30	
	One-Leg Dumbell Raise	10	35	1	10	35	
	One-Leg Dumbell Raise	8	40	1	8	40	
	One-Leg Dumbell Raise	6	45	2	6	45	
Abs	Incline Bent Leg Sit Ups	12	~	1	12	~	
	Incline Bent Leg Sit Ups	10	~	1	10	~	
	Incline Bent Leg Sit Ups	8	~	1	8	~	
	Incline Bent Leg Sit Ups	20	~	2	20	~	
Abs	Incline Leg Raises	12	~	1	12	~	
	Incline Leg Raises	10	~	1	10	~	
	Incline Leg Raises	8	~	1	8	~	
	Incline Leg Raises	20	~	2	20	~	

NOTES

Getting stronger with leg extensions.

Felt burn on the last set of sit ups of 20 reps.

Increase leg curls by 5 lbs per set next time.

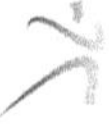

Workout A: Chest • Shoulders • Triceps

Daily Workout Progress Planner

Date:	Planned Start Time:	Actual Start Time:
Day:	Planned End Time:	Actual End Time:
Chest • Shoulders • Triceps	Estimated to Complete:	Total Time Taken:

		PLAN			ACTUAL		
Workout A	Exercise	Reps	Weight (lbs.)	Minutes Between Sets	Reps	Weight (lbs.)	NOTES
Chest		12		1			
		10		1			
		8		1			
		6		2			
Chest		12		1			
		10		1			
		8		1			
		6		2			
Shoulders		12		1			
		10		1			
		8		1			
		6		2			
Shoulders		12		1			
		10		1			
		8		1			
		6		2			
Triceps		12		1			
		10		1			
		8		1			
		6		2			
Triceps		12		1			
		10		1			
		8		1			
		6		2			

NOTES

Workout B: Back • Biceps • Forearms

Daily Workout Progress Planner

Date:	Planned Start Time:	Actual Start Time:
Day:	Planned End Time:	Actual End Time:
Back • Biceps • Forearms	Estimated to Complete:	Total Time Taken:

		PLAN			ACTUAL		
Workout B	Exercise	Reps	Weight (lbs.)	Minutes Between Sets	Reps	Weight (lbs.)	NOTES
Back		12		1			
		10		1			
		8		1			
		6		2			
Back		12		1			
		10		1			
		8		1			
		6		2			
Biceps		12		1			
		10		1			
		8		1			
		6		2			
Biceps		12		1			
		10		1			
		8		1			
		6		2			
Forearms		12		1			
		10		1			
		8		1			
		6		2			
Forearms		12		1			
		10		1			
		8		1			
		6		2			

NOTES

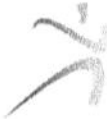

Workout C: Legs • Calves • Abs

Daily Workout Progress Planner

Date:	Planned Start Time:	Actual Start Time:
Day:	Planned End Time:	Actual End Time:
Legs • Calves • Abs	Estimated to Complete:	Total Time Taken:

		PLAN			ACTUAL		
Workout C	**Exercise**	**Reps**	**Weight (lbs.)**	**Minutes Between Sets**	**Reps**	**Weight (lbs.)**	**NOTES**
Legs		12		1			
		10		1			
		8		1			
		6		2			
Legs		12		1			
		10		1			
		8		1			
		6		2			
Calves		12		1			
		10		1			
		8		1			
		6		2			
Calves		12		1			
		10		1			
		8		1			
		6		2			
Abs		12		1			
		10		1			
		8		1			
		6		2			
Abs		12		1			
		10		1			
		8		1			
		6		2			

NOTES

The Exercise Guide

Preliminary Stretching Exercises

CHEST Stretch

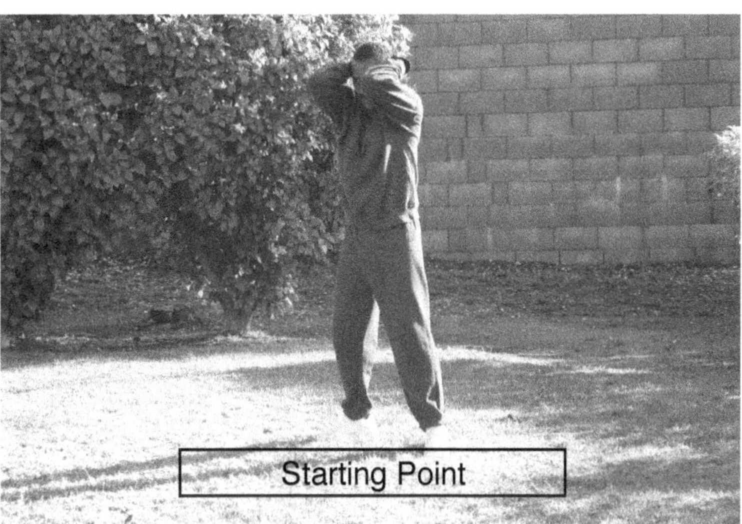

"What you can do, or dream you can do, begin it; boldness has genius, power and magic in it."–Johann von Goethe

Starting Position: Stand and interlock your fingers behind your head with your elbows pointed in front of you.

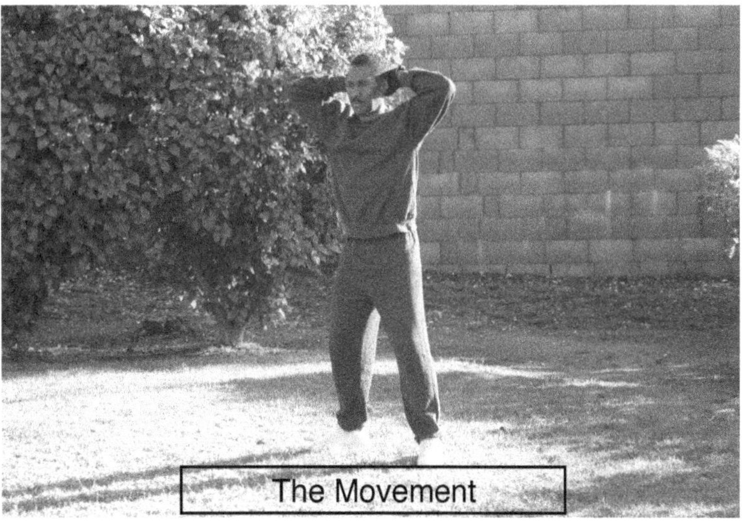

The Exercise: Squeeze your shoulder blades together rotating your elbows to the sides. Hold this stretch for 20 seconds.

Preliminary Stretching Exercises

LAT Stretch

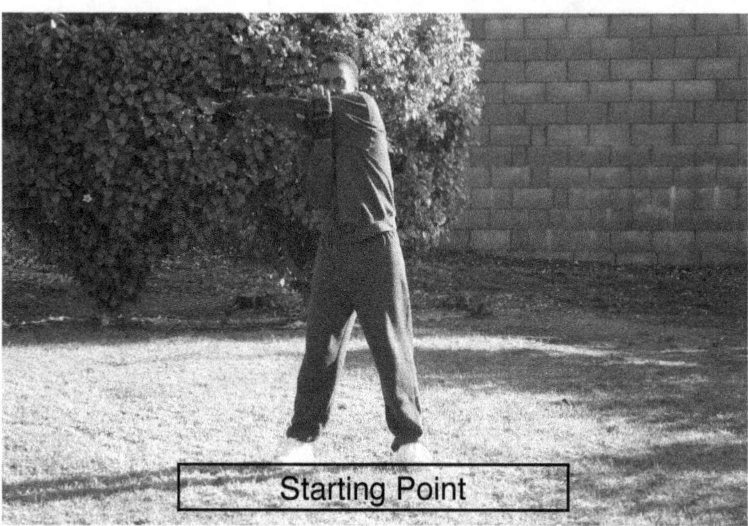

Starting Point

Starting Position: Stand with feet shoulder-width apart. Cross your left arm over your chest parallel to the ground. Grasp your left elbow with your right forearm.

"Beware of dissipating your powers; strive constantly to concentrate them."–Johann von Goethe

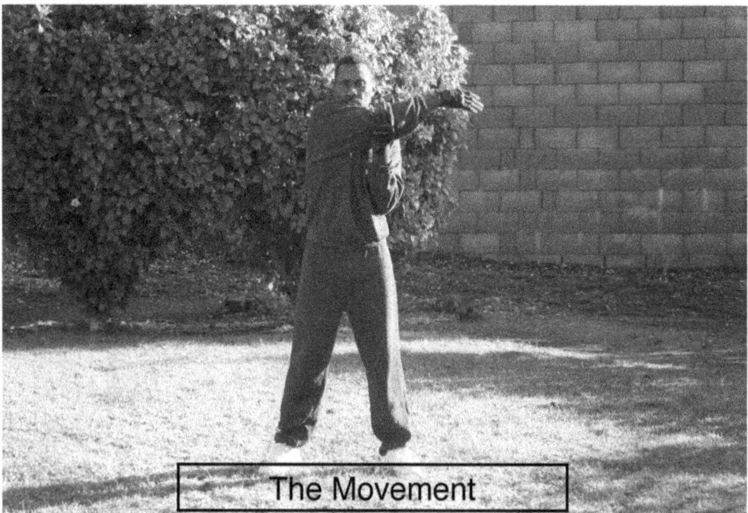

The Movement

The Exercise: Pull on your elbow until you feel a moderate stretch in your upper lat region. Hold this stretch for 20 seconds, and switch sides and repeat for 20 seconds.

Preliminary Stretching Exercises

SHOULDER Stretch

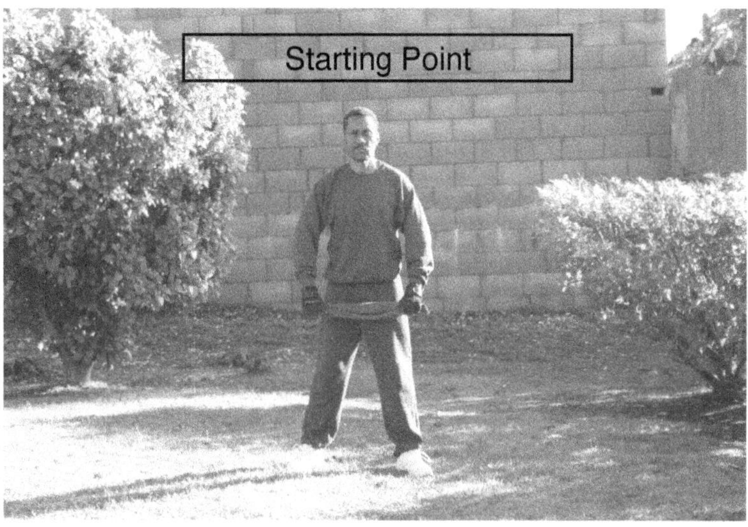

Starting Position: Stand with feet shoulder-width apart. Hold a towel in front of you with your arms at your sides.

"We will either find a way, or make one."–Hannibal

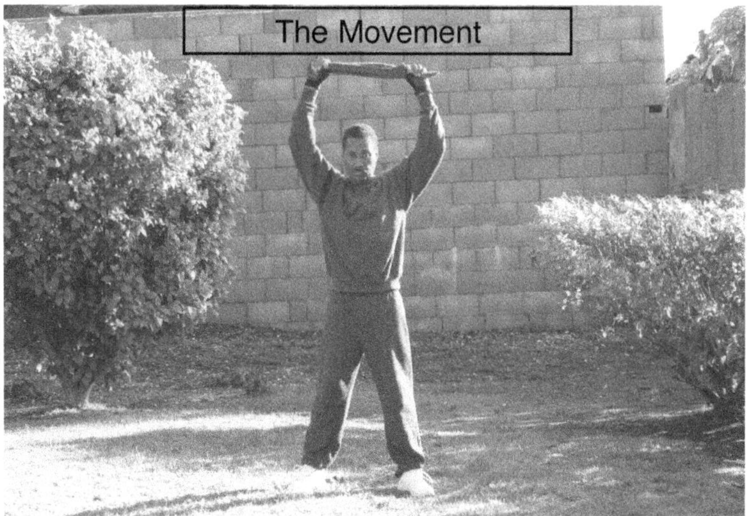

The Exercise: Lift your arms overhead keeping your elbows locked; spread your arms apart as far as possible with the towel taut. Hold this stretch for 20 seconds.

Preliminary Stretching Exercises

TORSO Stretch

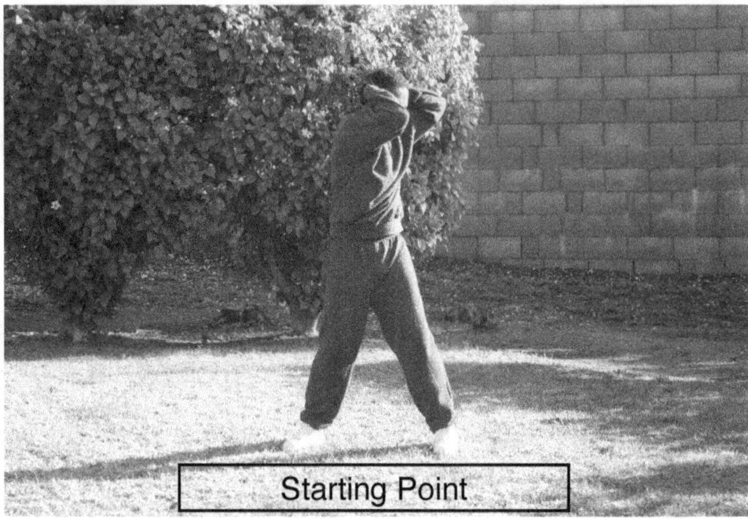

Starting Point

Starting Position: Stand with your fingers interlaced behind your head.

"Belief is the only door through which the power of God can flow."–Charles Prosper

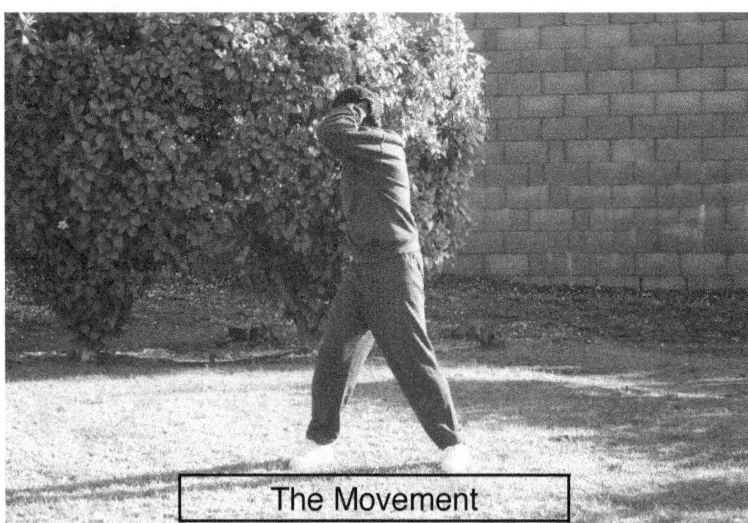

The Movement

The Exercise: Rotate your torso all the way to the right when you feel a stretch in your waist, hold this stretch for 20 seconds, then switch sides and repeat for 20 seconds.

Preliminary Stretching Exercises

QUADRICEPS Stretch

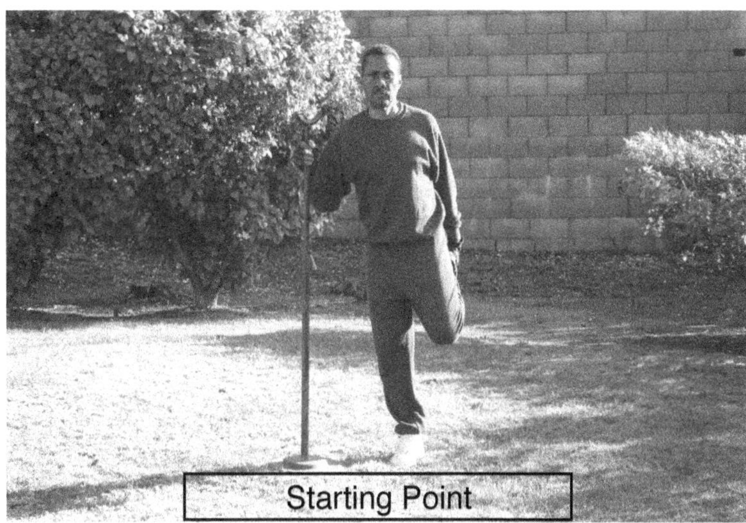

Starting Point

The Exercise: Stand upright, arms at side, feet together. Grasp your left foot in your left hand.

"Results are what you expect; consequences are what you get."–Anonymous

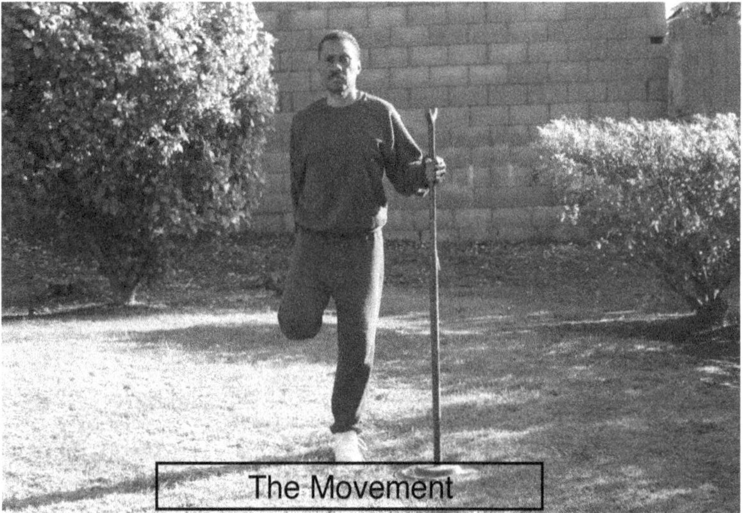

The Movement

The Exercise: Pull until you feel a moderate stretch. Hold for 20 seconds. Then switch legs.

Workout A - Chest

Bench Press

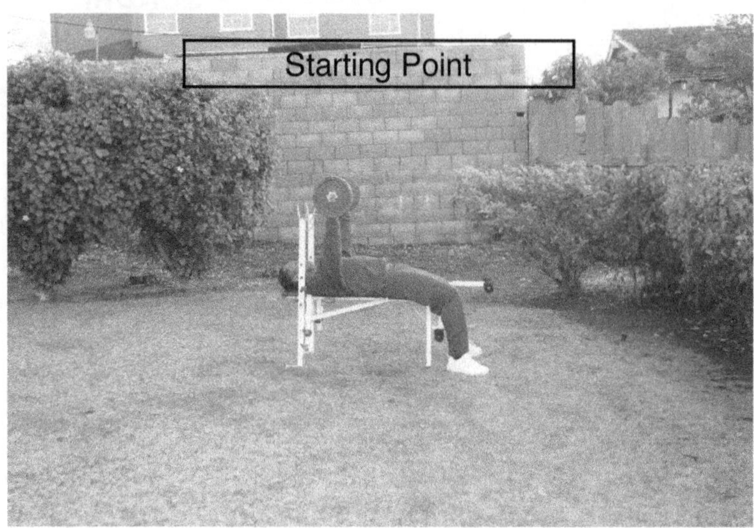

Starting Position: Lie on your bench and keep your feet flat on the floor. Grab a long barbell, shoulder-width grip. Lift up so that it is in line with your shoulders.

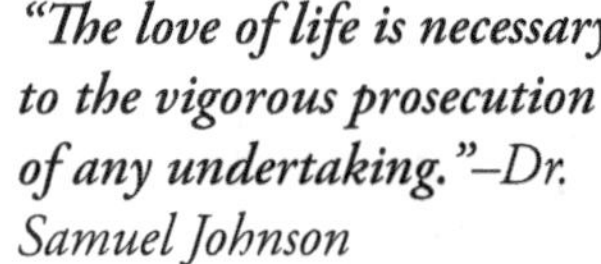
"The love of life is necessary to the vigorous prosecution of any undertaking."–Dr. Samuel Johnson

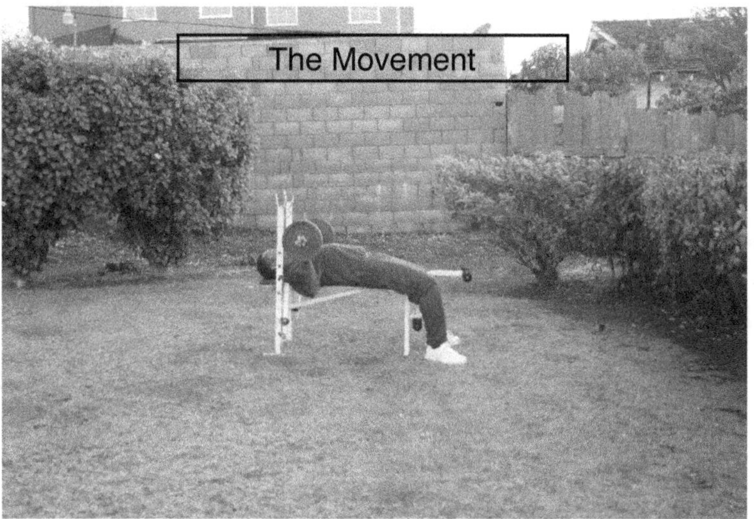

The Exercise: Lower the barbell to your chest, even with your nipple-line. Keep elbow back and your chest held high with your back slightly arched. Keep your head and hips on the bench. Exhale as you push up.

Workout A - Chest

Dumbbell Bench Press

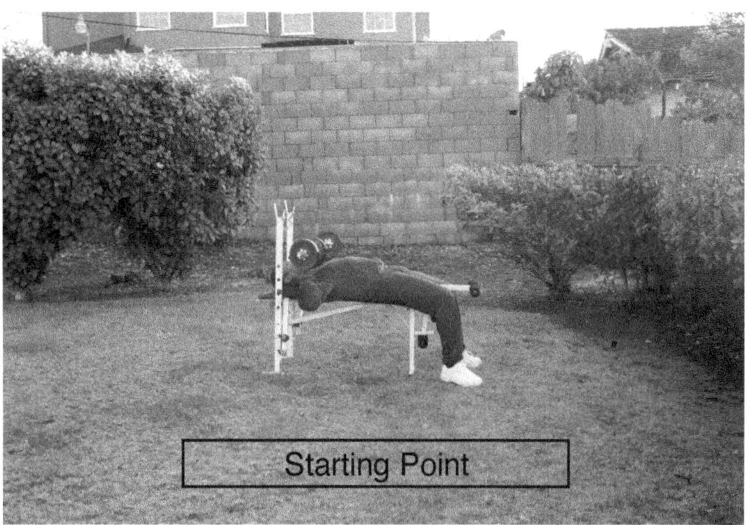

Starting Point

Starting Position: Grab a pair of dumbbells. Lie on your bench with feet flat on the floor. Hold the two dumbbells just above your shoulders with your palms facing your feet and your elbows pointing out.

"It wasn't raining when Noah built the ark."–Howard Ruff

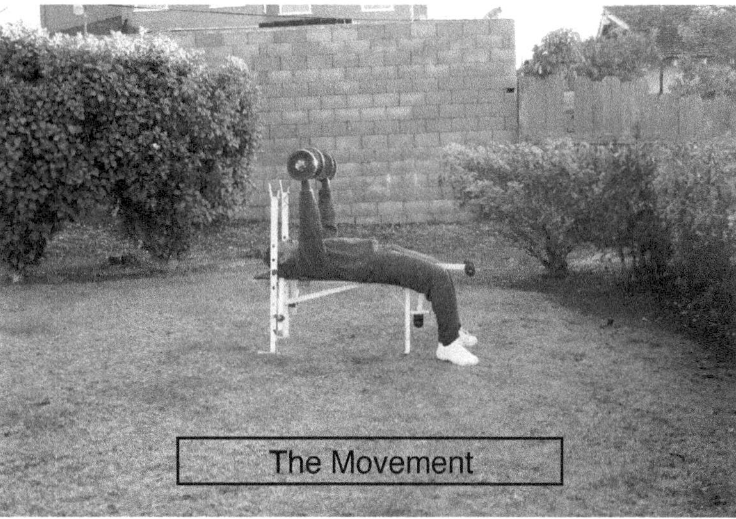

The Movement

The Exercise: Push the weights up until your elbows lock then slowly lower the dumbbells back to your shoulders. Make sure that the path of the dumbbells follow a straight line over your collarbone area - not over your face area.

Workout A - Chest

Inclined Bench Press

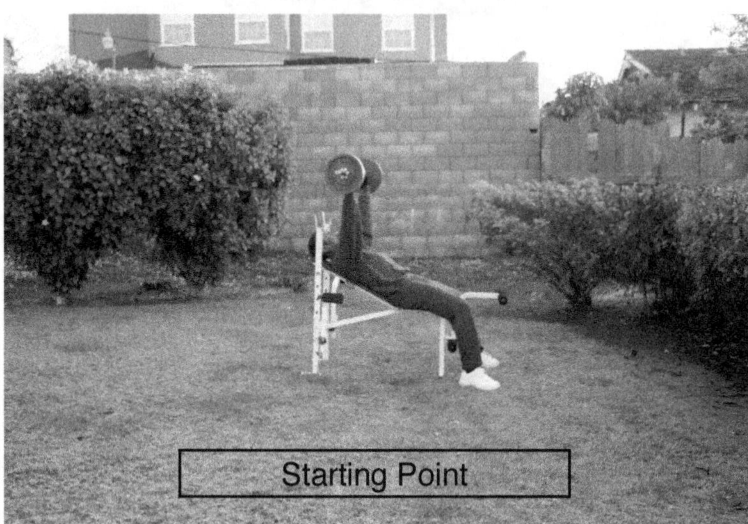

Starting Point

Starting Position: On an inclined bench, rest your back. Using a shoulder width grip, take the long barbell off of the rack.

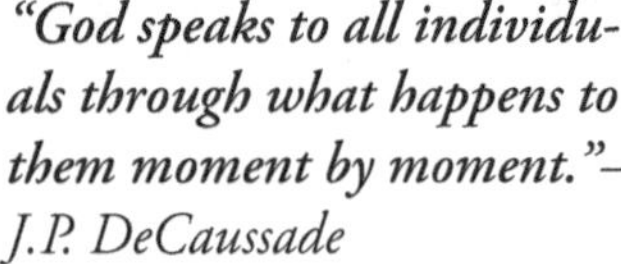

"God speaks to all individuals through what happens to them moment by moment."– J.P. DeCaussade

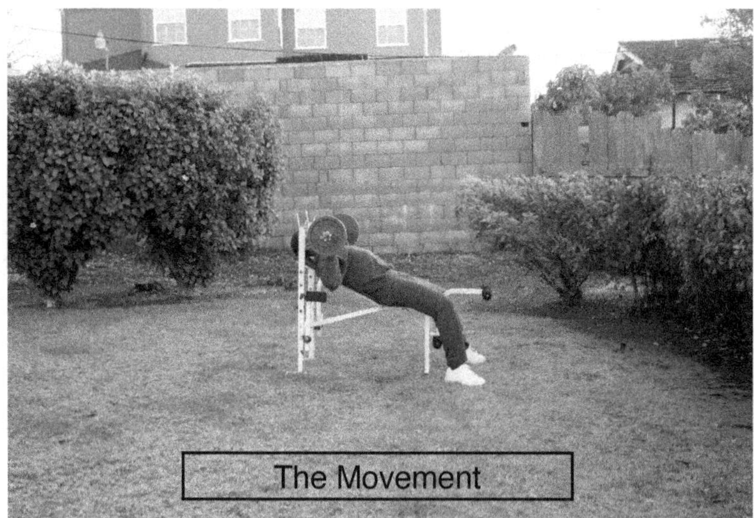

The Movement

The Exercise: Lower the bar down to your upper chest. Exhale as you push the bar back to your starting position. Keep head and hips on bench, slightly arching your back. When you lower the bar, aim for your upper chest.

 www.fitfastatanyage.com www.fitfastatanyage.com

Workout A - Chest

Flat Dumbbell Flyes

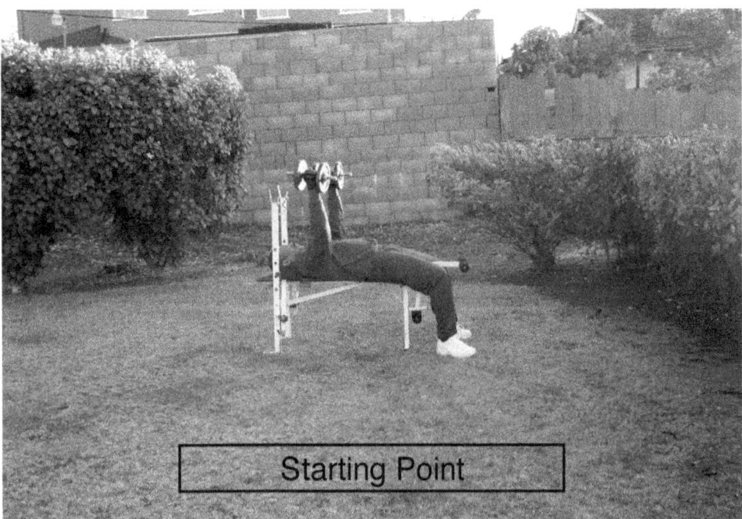

Starting Point

Starting Position: Lying down on a bench, extend two dumbbells above your head, at arm's length slightly touching each other with palms facing inward and elbows slightly bent throughout the entire exercise.

"God hasn't called me to be successful. He's called me to be faithful."–Mother Teresa

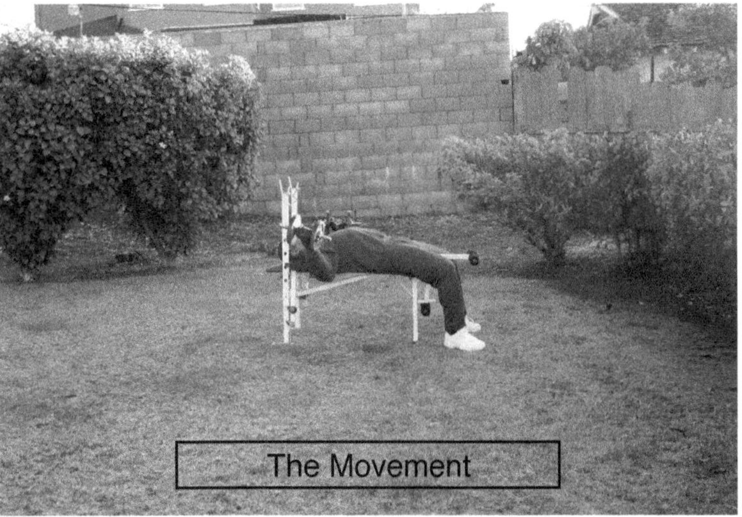

The Movement

The Exercise: Lower carefully the two dumbbells, elbows locked, in a semicircle pattern until they are about even with the sides of your chest. Keep your chest high and back slightly arched. Exhale as you return them to the starting point above your body again.

Workout A - Chest

Inclined Dumbbell Flyes

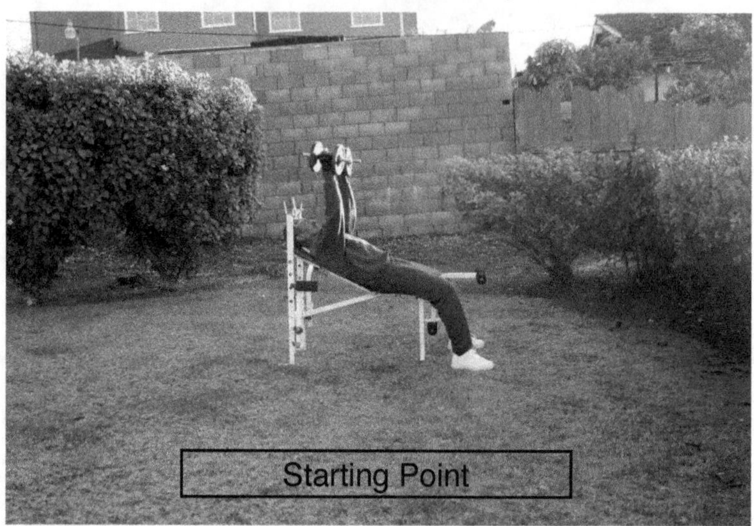

Starting Point

Starting Position: With two light dumbbells above your head, extended up at arm's length, slightly touching each other with palms facing inward. (The incline bench shifts the workout to the upper chest muscles.)

"A consciousness of God releases the greatest power of all."–Science of Mind

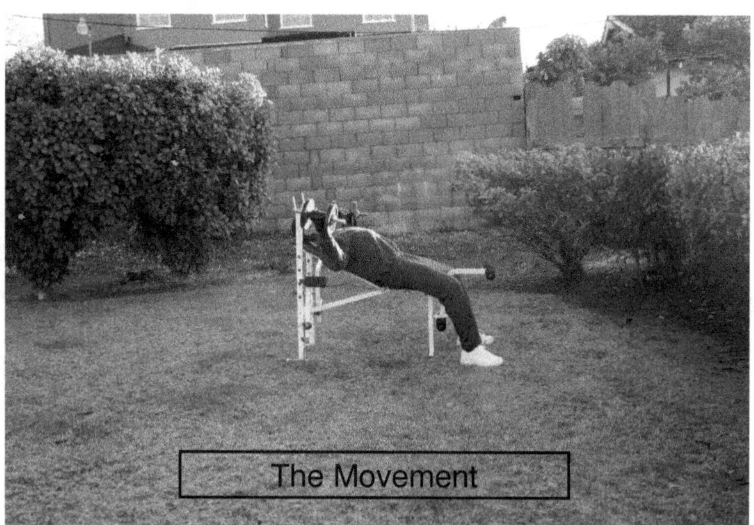

The Movement

The Exercise: Lower your weights out and to each sides of your chest until they are about even with the chest. With chest high and your back slightly arched, return to the starting position above as you exhale upon completion of each movement.

Workout A - Chest

Floor Push-Ups

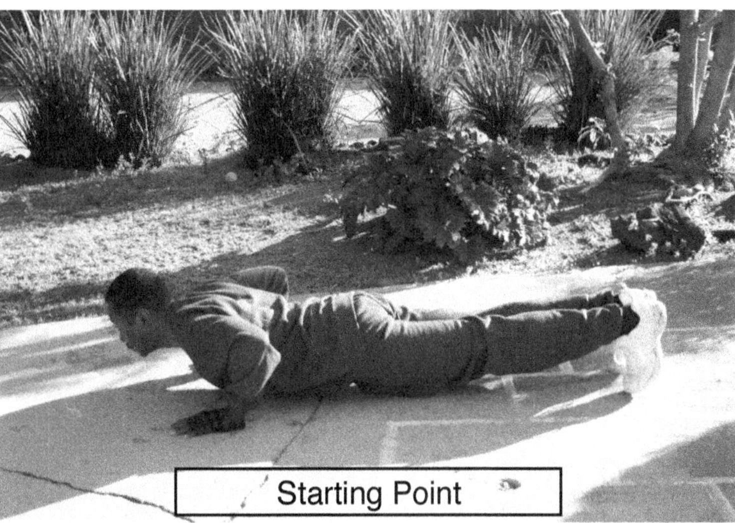

Starting Point

Starting Position: Lie face down with your arms straight and palms flat on the floor with your hands should-width apart. Hold your feet together or very slightly spread.

"Many of life's failures are men who did not realize how close they were to success when they gave up."–Thomas Alva Edison

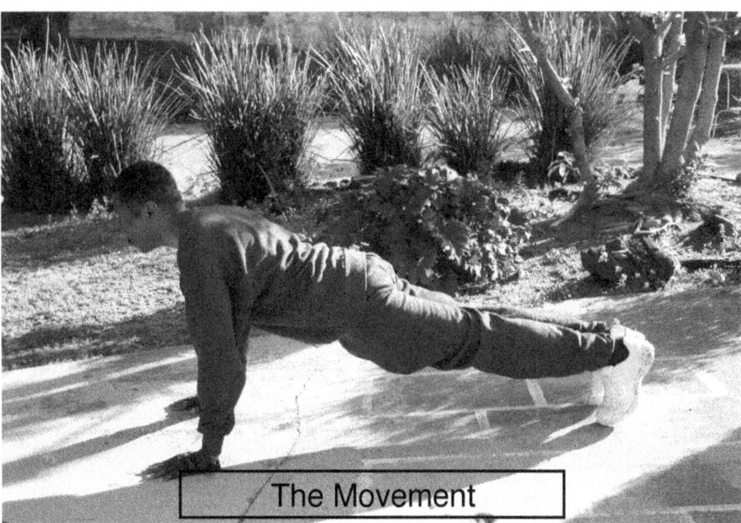

The Movement

The Exercise: Push yourself to an arms-extended position and exhale as you complete the movement.

Workout A - Shoulders

Seated Barbell Press

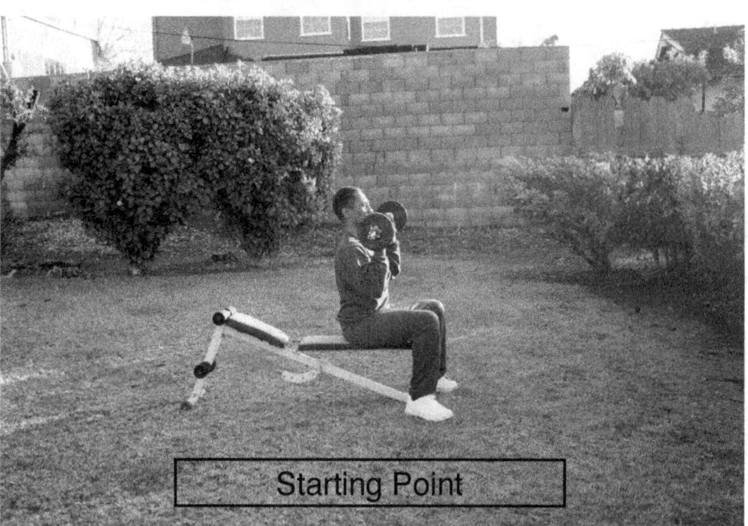

Starting Point

Starting Position: On the end of a bench, gently sit down. Lift the barbell up to your shoulders. Keep your eyes on the upward and downward movement of the barbell to avoid from hitting your head.

"We carry with us the wonders we seek without us."–Sir Thomas Browne

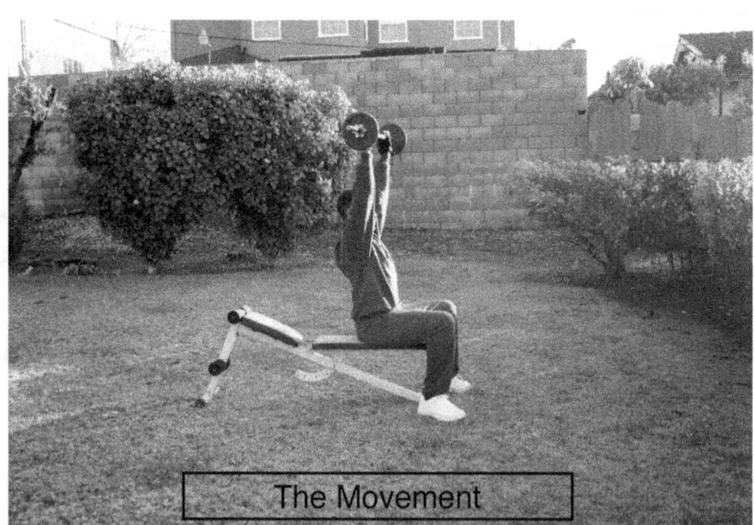

The Movement

The Exercise: Press the barbell over your head while keeping your elbows in. Do not lock your elbows at the top of the move. Exhale as you slowly lower the barbell.

Workout A - Shoulders

Seated Dumbbell Press

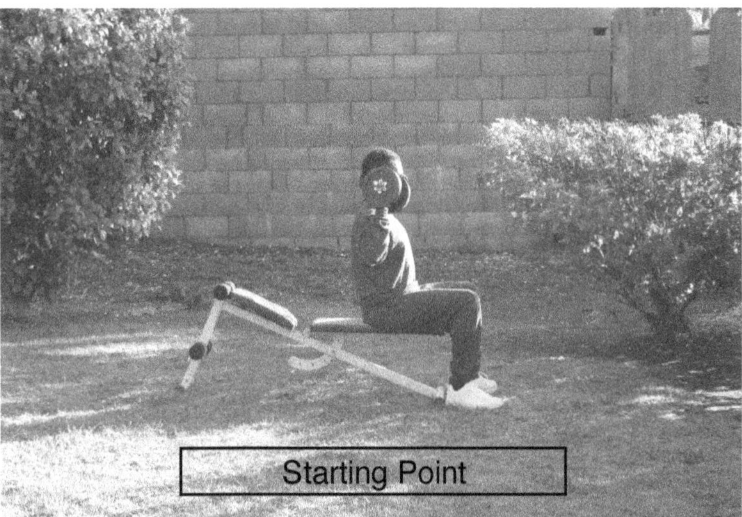

Starting Point

"Forgiveness is the sweetest revenge."–Isaac Friedmann

Starting Position: Lift two dumbbells to your shoulders with your palms facing outward. Put your feet firmly on the floor. Raise your chest and head up and keep your back straight.

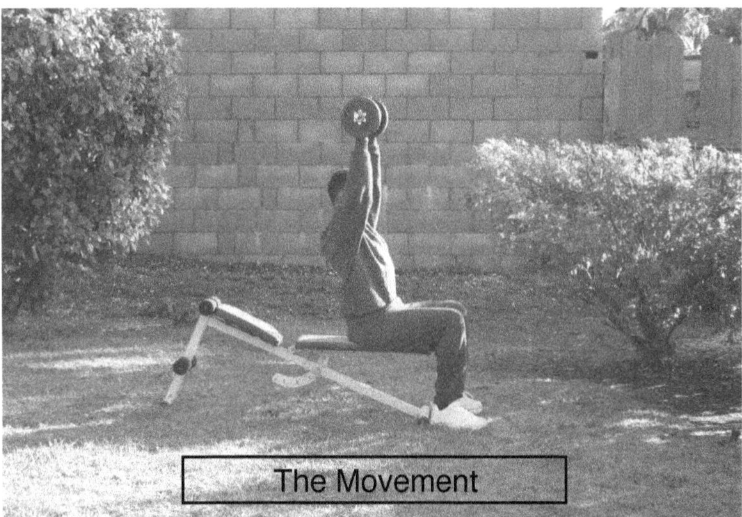

The Movement

The Exercise: Lift the two dumbbells overhead to arm's length while keeping your elbows outwards. Lower them again to the starting position. Exhale as you lower the weights.

Workout A - Shoulders

Dumbbell Side Raises

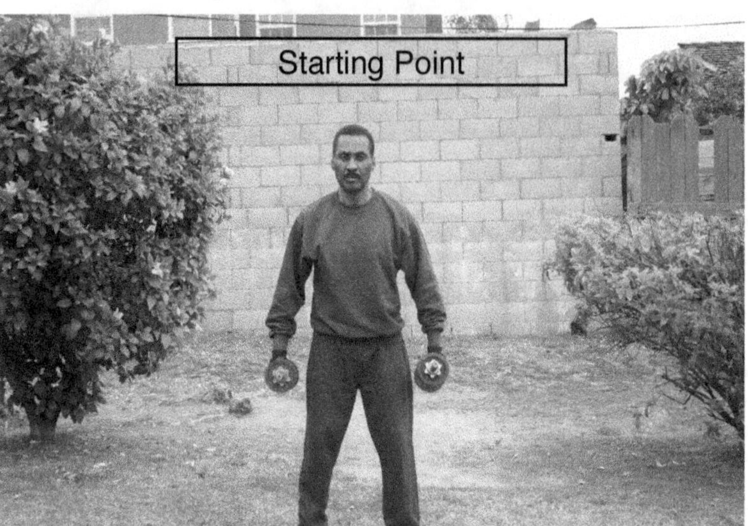

Starting Position: Standing shoulder's width apart, with two dumbbells held in front of your thighs, palms facing inward. Now you may bend forward slightly at the waist to begin the movement.

"If you really want to do something, you'll find a way; if you don't, you'll find an excuse."–Anonymous

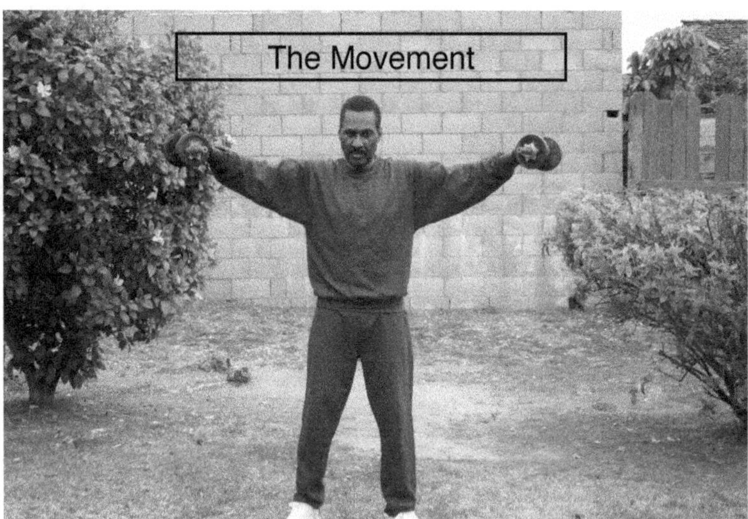

The Exercise: Raise the dumbbells in a smooth and controlled manner up and out towards your sides. Inhale as you lift them, and exhale as you lower them. Raise the dumbbells slightly higher than shoulders' level, and in a controlled fashion lower them back down.

Workout A - Shoulders

Bent-Over Side Raises

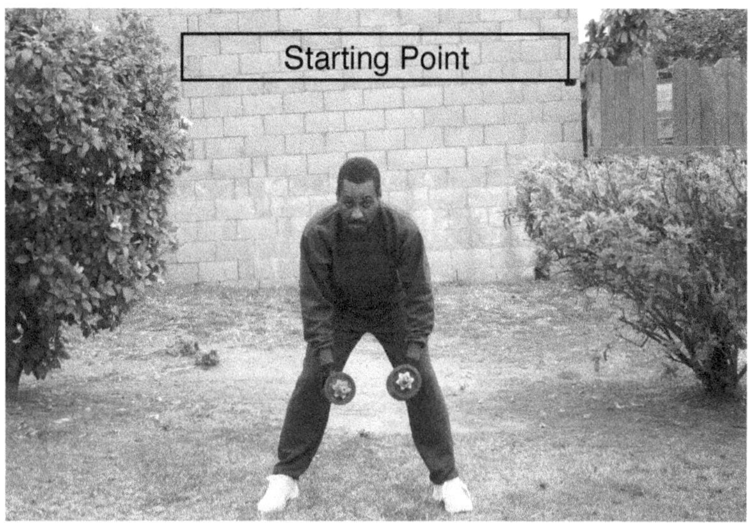

Starting Position: Place your feet shoulder's width apart and with a dumbbell in each hand, bend forward carefully at the waist with you upper body parallel to the floor with your arms hanging straight down and the palms facing each other.

"Faith is to believe what we do not see; the reward of this faith is to see what we believe."–Saint Augustine

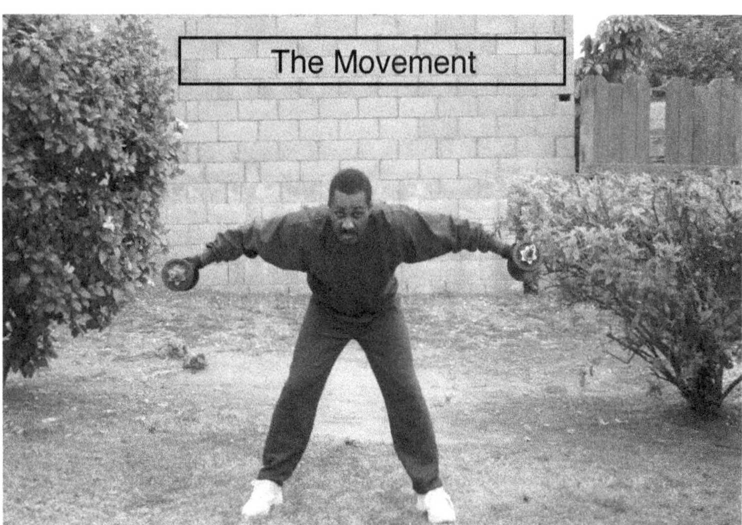

The Exercise: Pulling your arms apart while moving your elbows up, raise the dumbbells upwards. Be careful not to raise your torso as you lift the weights, and do not bend down and lean your torso below a straight parallel line to the floor. Keep your torso stationary.

Workout A - Shoulders

Standing Barbell Press

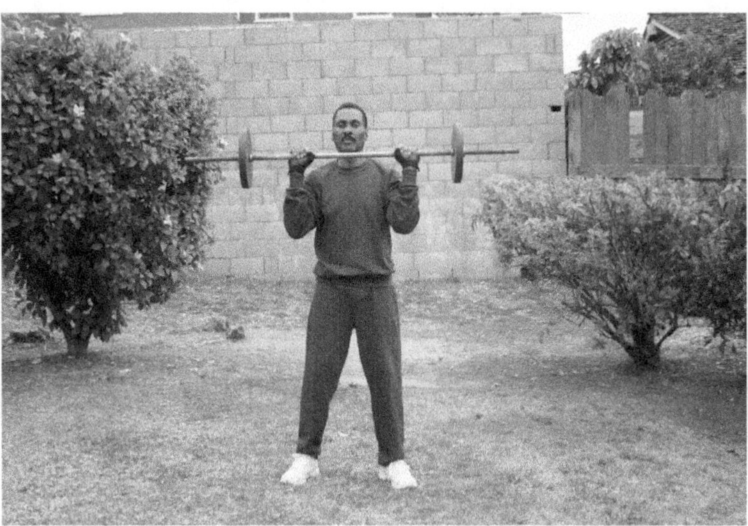

Starting Position: With your feet placed shoulder-width apart, bend your knees slightly while keeping your back straight being careful not to arch it as you lift. Grip the barbell a little broader than shoulder-width, starting with it just above your collarbone.

"We cannot direct the wind, but we can adjust the sails."–Bertha Calloway

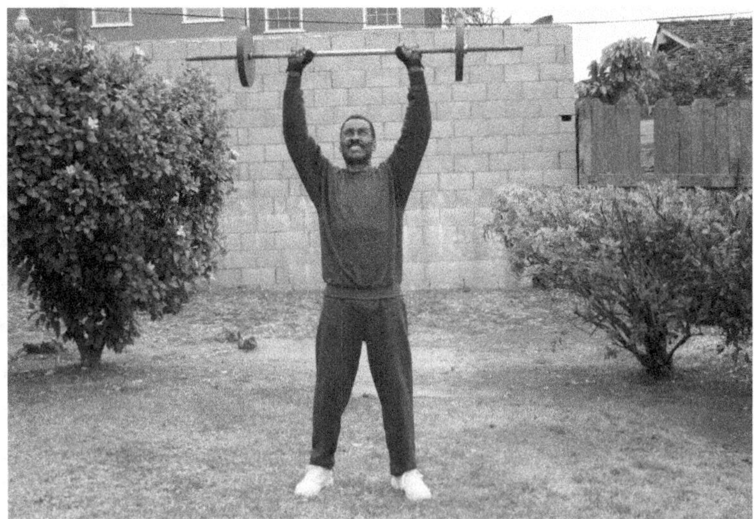

The Exercise: Push the barbell up and over your head. The most important thing is to not arch your back as you press the barbell to avoid lower back injury. If you are having to arch too much to press the weight upwards, then you probably need to reduce the weight.

Workout A - Triceps

Lying Barbell Triceps Extensions

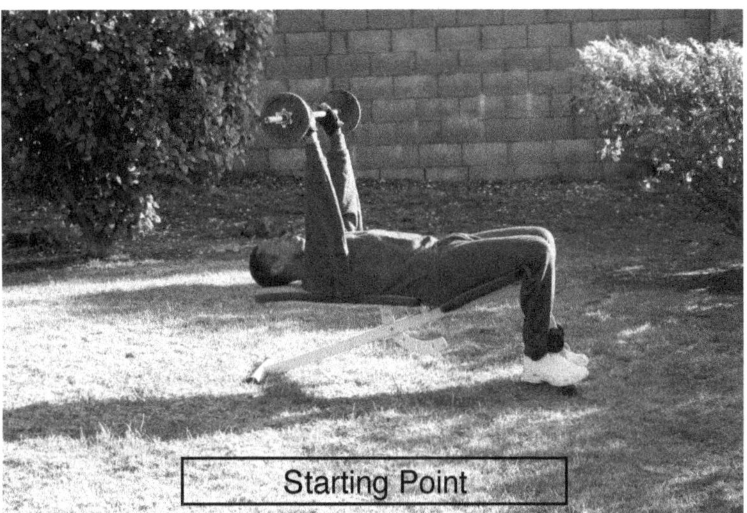

Starting Point

Starting Position: Pick up your barbell, and lie on your workout bench. With your hands about a foot apart on the bar, extend the barbell up to arm's length above your shoulder line.

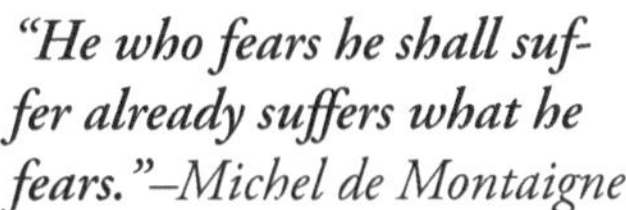

"He who fears he shall suffer already suffers what he fears."–Michel de Montaigne

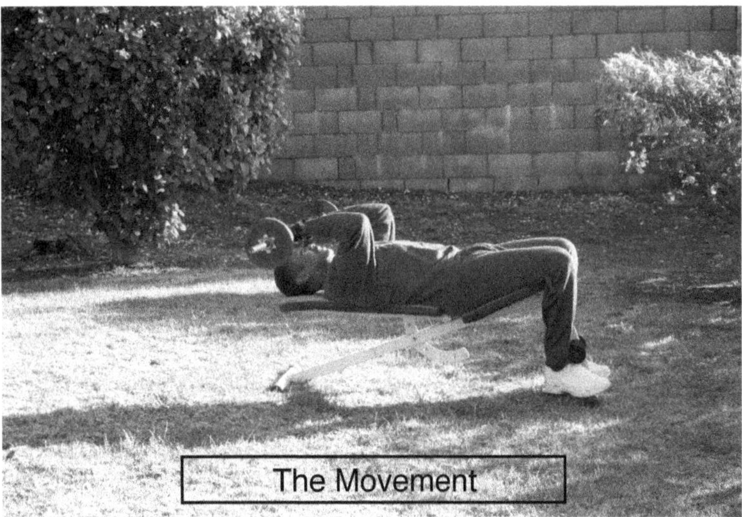

The Movement

The Exercise: Lower carefully the barbell just above your forehead with your elbows pointing to the ceiling. Press the barbell back to your starting position and exhale as you return. Lower the bar carefully so that you don't bop yourself in the head.

Workout A - Triceps

Overhead Dumbbell Triceps Extension

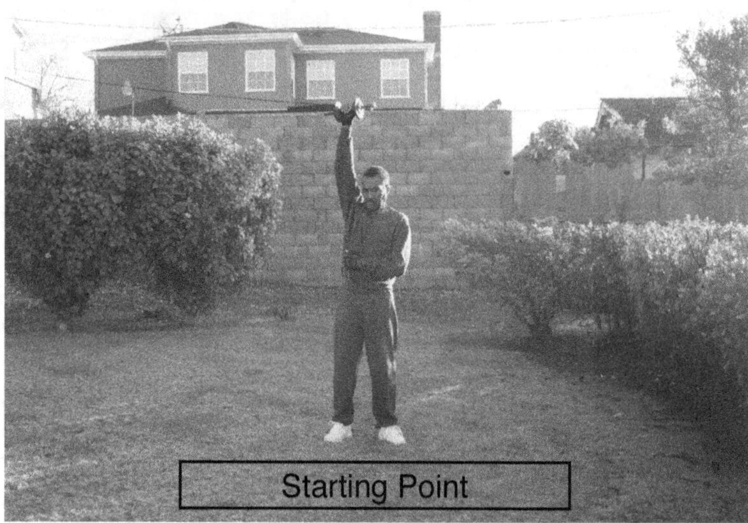

Starting Point

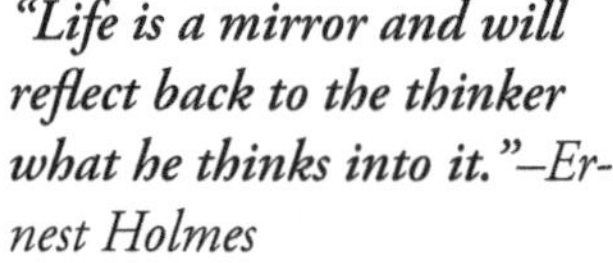

"Life is a mirror and will reflect back to the thinker what he thinks into it."–Ernest Holmes

Starting Position: Pick up a dumbbell in one hand and lift it overhead. (This exercise may be done seated or standing.) While seated you are forced to exercise more control.

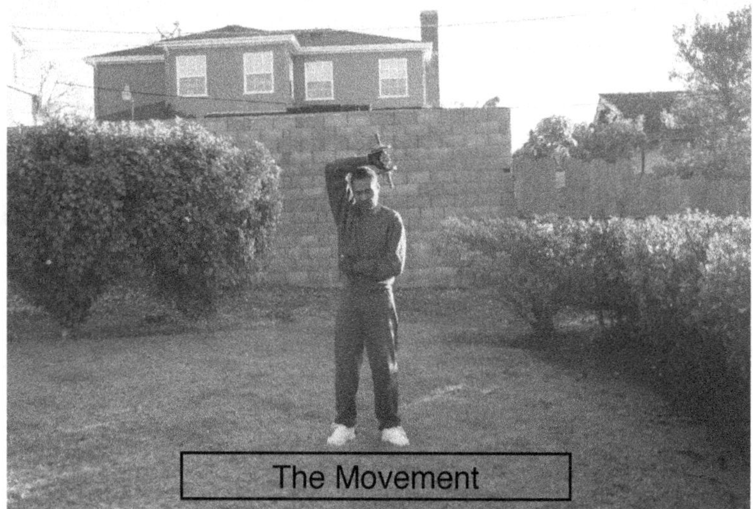

The Movement

The Exercise: Slowly lower the dumbbell behind your head as far as you can comfortably go. Return to starting point exhaling as you do. Be sure to keep your upper arms close to the side of your head and point your elbows up to the ceiling.

Workout A - Triceps

Bench Dips

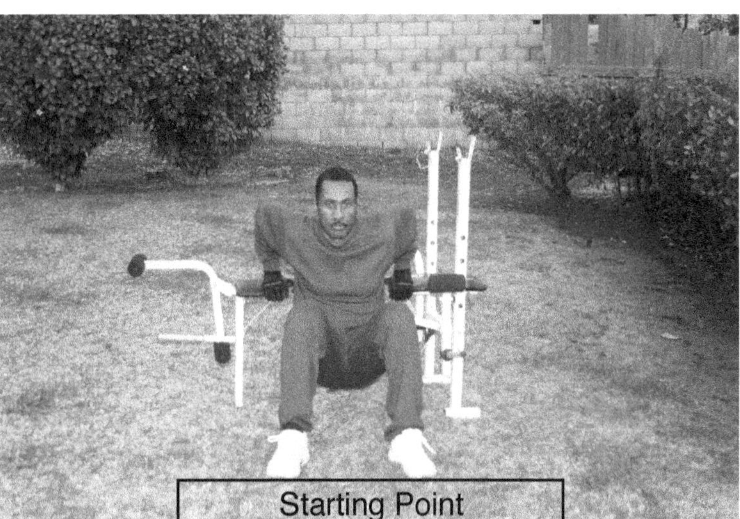

Starting Point

Starting Position: With your hands facing forward and your palms placed flat, grip the edge of a bench at shoulders-width. Place your feet together on the floor extending them out as far as possible. Now, slide your backside off of the bench.

"Our minds can shape the way a thing will be because we act according to our expectation."–Federico Fellini

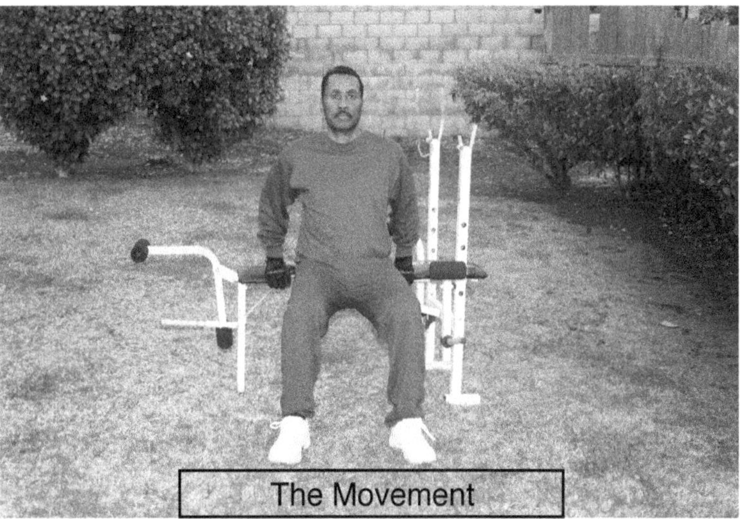

The Movement

The Exercise: Keeping your hips relatively close to the bench and while keeping your elbows locked, lower you body until your upper arms are parallel to the floor. Now push yourself back up to the starting position.

Workout A - Triceps

Standing Dumbbell Triceps Extentions

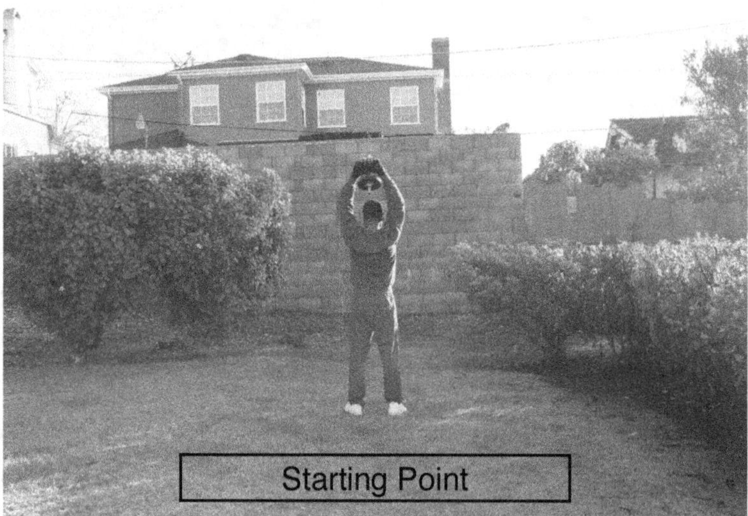

Starting Point

Starting Position: Find a dumbbell which has collars to hold the weights on firmly. With feet shoulder-width apart and knees slightly bent, grab one end of a dumbbell with both hands and raise it above. The inside end plate will rest on your palms-up position; thumbs will touch.

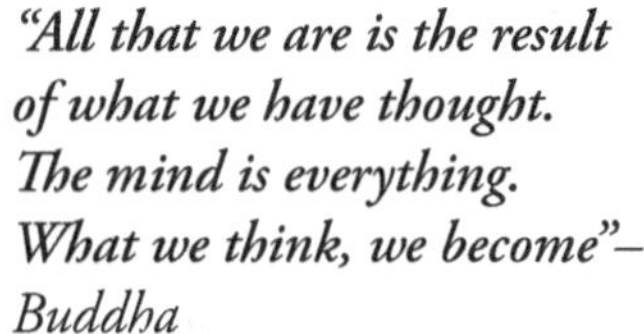

"All that we are is the result of what we have thought. The mind is everything. What we think, we become"– *Buddha*

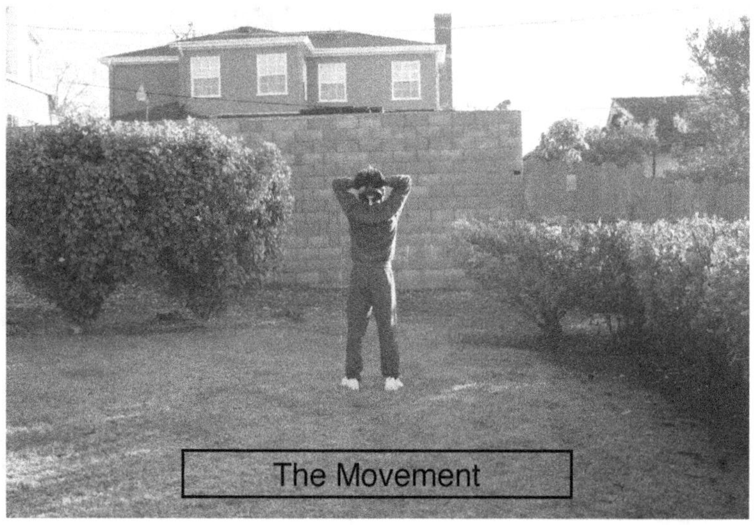

The Movement

The Exercise: Keeping your elbows pointed up, slowly lower the dumbbell behind the head, keeping your elbows close to your head. Lower the weight until you feel a stretch in your triceps muscle. Lift up again until your arms are locked out over your head.

Workout A - Triceps

Lying Dumbbell Triceps Extentions

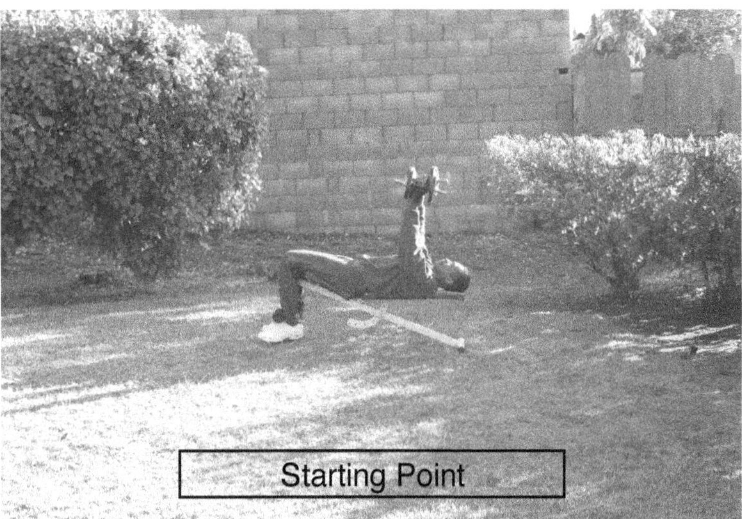
Starting Point

Starting Position: With a dumbbell in each hand, lie down flat on a workout bench with your arms extending above your head; you should be able to look straight up at each dumbbell, and your palms should be facing each other.

"God will help you if you try, and you can if you think you can."–Anne Delaney Peale

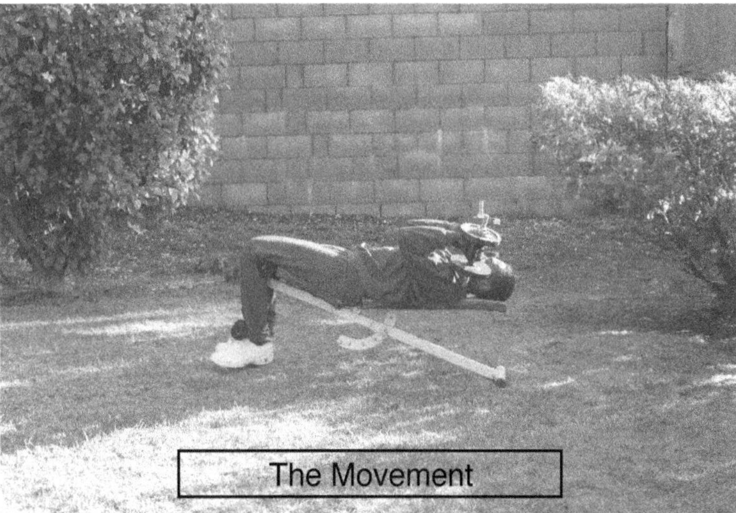
The Movement

The Exercise: While keeping your elbows pointed up and not back, keep your upper arms stationary. You must slowly lower your dumbbells at the elbows – down towards your shoulders. Just be sure not to allow your elbows to fly – outwards; pull them in and up.

Workout B - Back

Underhand Chin-Ups

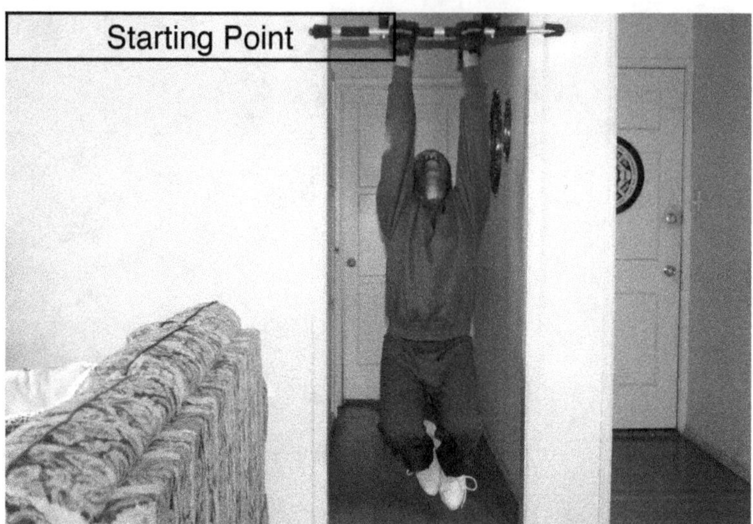

Starting Position: Grab a doorway chinning bar with a palms-facing-you grip. Place hands about shoulder-width apart. Lift your feet off the ground and slightly arch your back and lean back a bit.

"Nothing is permanent but change."–Heraclitus

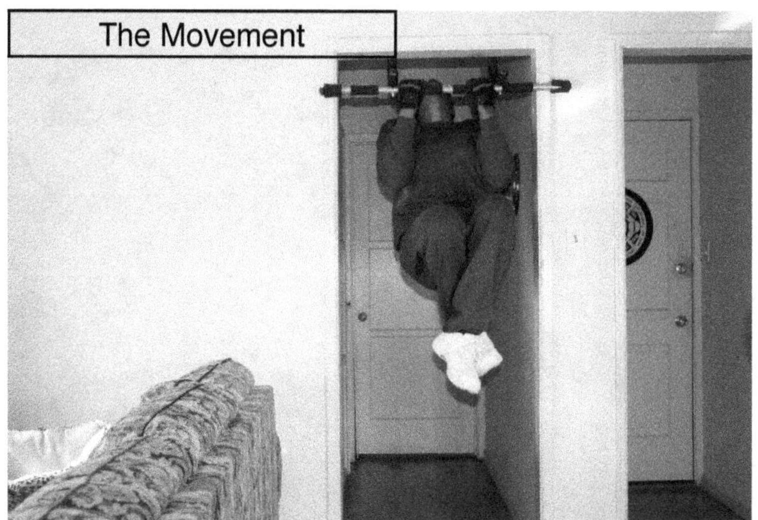

The Exercise: Pull yourself up as high as you can inhaling as you do. (This is an advanced exercise and requires good upper body strength.) I used to call them 3-inch chin-ups until I could make it up all of the way. Be patient and do as many of the reps that you can.

Workout B - Back

Bent-Over Barbell Row

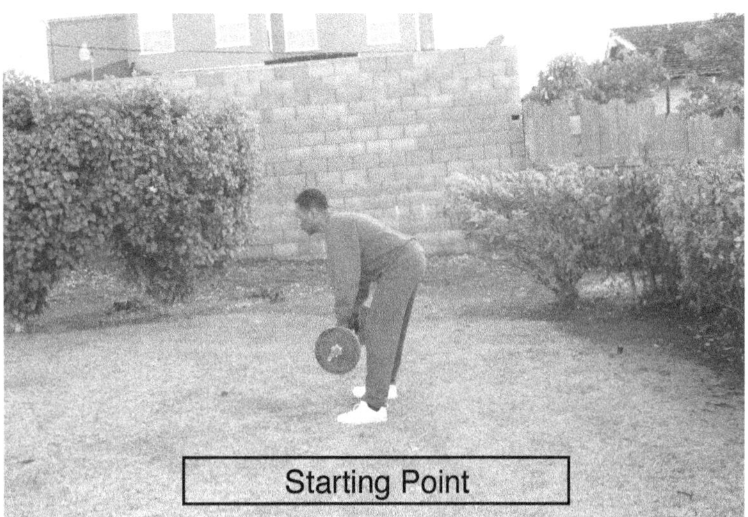

Starting Point

Starting Position: With your feet shoulder-width apart, stand in front of a barbell. Making sure your back is straight and parallel to the floor, bend over and grab the barbell. Keep your head up and your legs slightly bent.

"Arriving at one goal is the starting point of another."– John Dewey

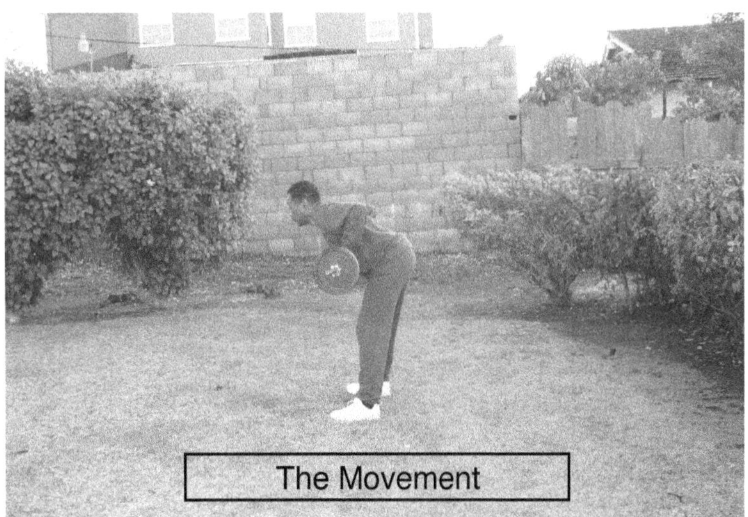

The Movement

The Exercise: As you pull the barbell upwards towards your lower chest, inhale. Then exhale as you lower it. Do not arch your back forward and downward toward the floor; keep it straight. Make sure you have stretched and that your lower back is warmed up.

Workout B - Back

Bent-Over Dumbell Row

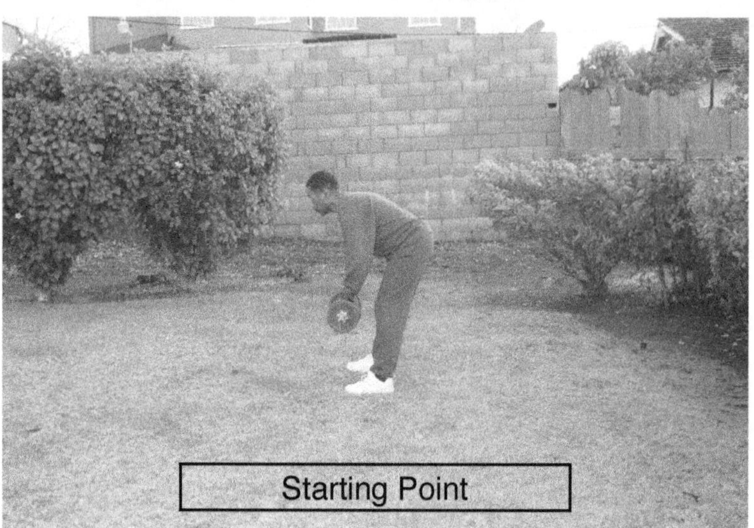

Starting Point

Starting Position: Place your feet together, and bend over and grab each of two dumbbells that are besides your feet. Keep your legs slightly bent, back straight and your head up. (From the angle of this photo, it is difficult to see the two dumbbells, but there are indeed one in each of my hands.)

"This above all: to thine own self be true."–William Shakespeare

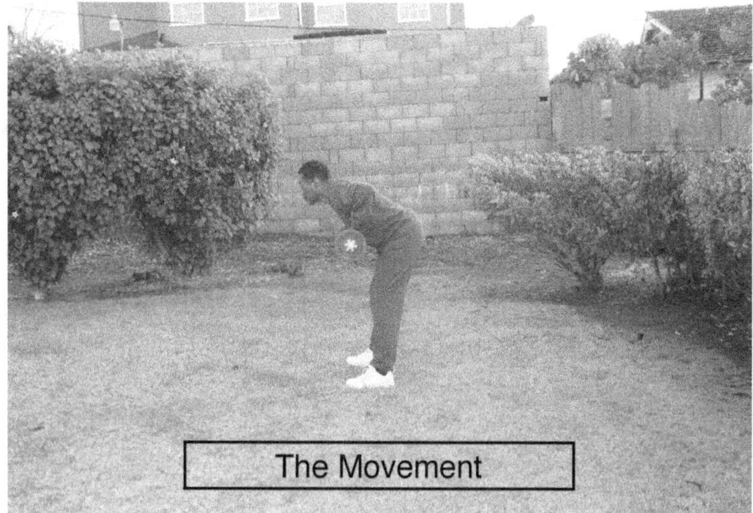

The Movement

The Exercise: Pull the dumbbells up to the sides of your chest and inhale while keeping your head up. Exhale as you lower them carefully to knee level again.

Workout B - Back

One-Arm Dumbell Row

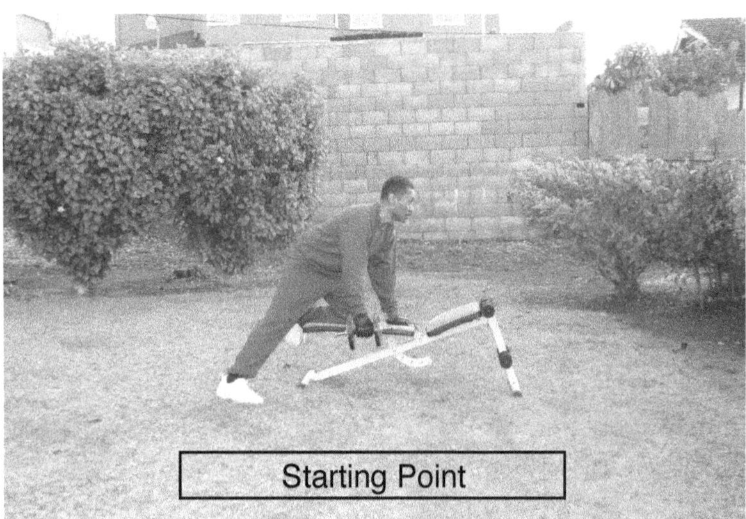
Starting Point

Starting Position: Place your left knee on a bench with your right leg stretched out. Grab the dumbbell with your right hand, the same side as the straight leg, with a "palms-in" grip. Place your left hand on the bench to brace and stabilize your movement.

"We fear the thing we want the most."–Dr. Robert Anthony

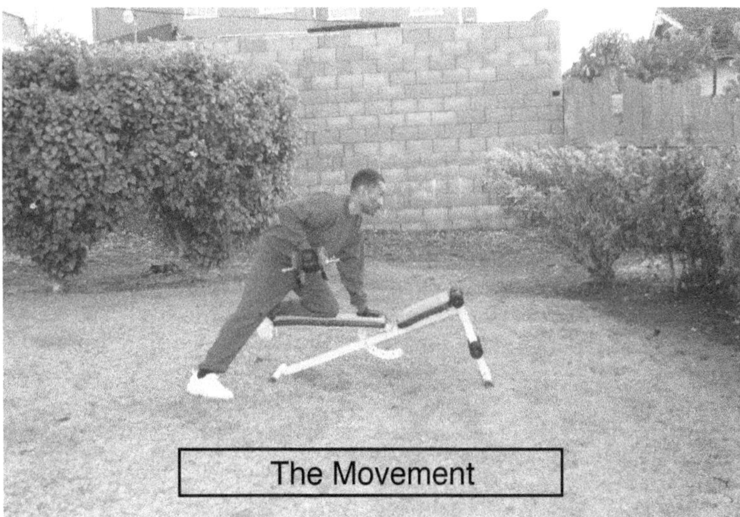
The Movement

The Exercise: Pull the dumbbell up as your arm moves up and your elbow back bringing the weight up to the side of your chest. Inhale as you lift. Now carefully lower the dumbbell, while exhaling, back to your starting point.

Workout B - Back

Dumbbell Deadlift

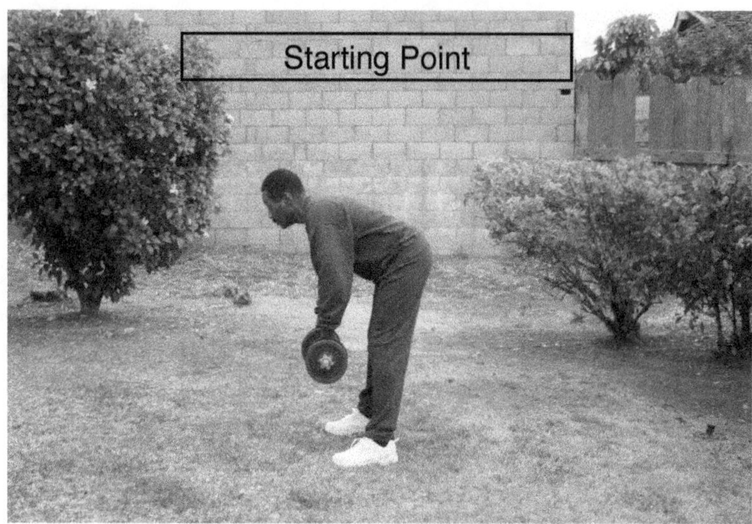

Starting Position: Standing with your feet about 10 inches apart, bend down at the waist and grasp your dumbbells. Keep your back straight, knees slightly bent and your head up.

"Be bold, and mighty forces will come to your aide."–Basil King

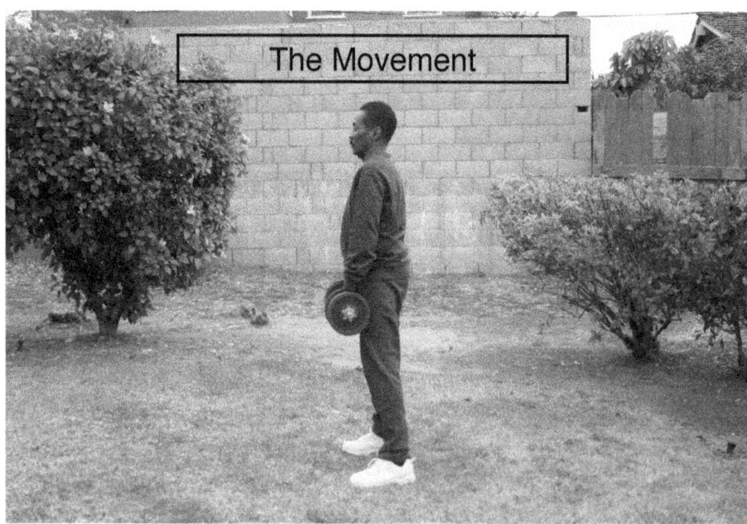

The Exercise: Stand back with your dumbbells in your hands, locking out your elbows while keeping your weights as close to your body as you can. Think about pushing your hips forward as you pick up the dumbbells.

Workout B - Back

Barbell Deadlift

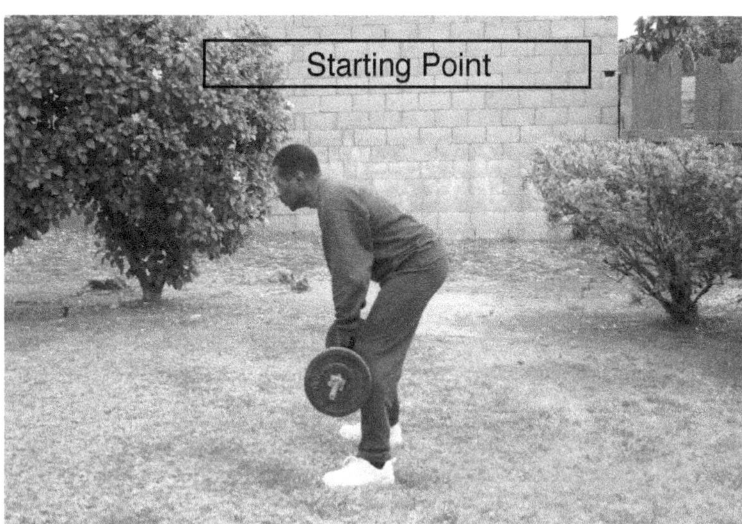

Starting Position: With your feet shoulder-width apart, bend your knees first, bend over and grasp the bar with an overhand grip while keeping your back straight and your head up.

"Pray that success will not come any faster than you are able to endure it."–Elbert Hubbard

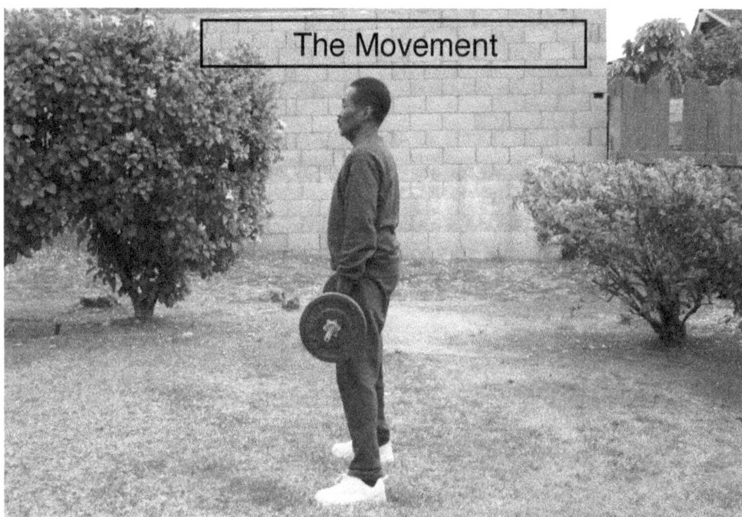

The Exercise: As you carefully move back up erect, keep the bar as close to your legs as possible. Lower the barbell down carefully to your starting point again. (Do not lower the barbell with your legs locked: doing this can cause injury to your lower back.)

Workout B - Arms (Biceps)

Standing Barbell Curl

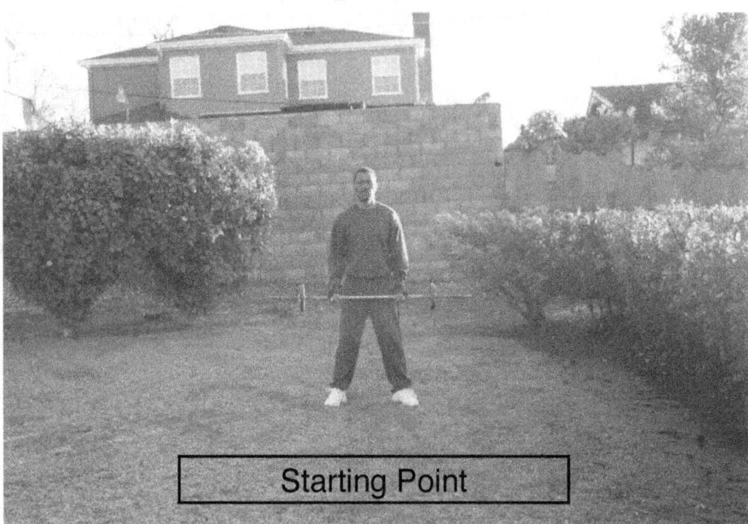

Starting Point

Starting Position: With your hands shoulder-width on the barbell, stand and hold the barbell at arm's length as it rests on your upper thighs.

"Love, and do what you like."–Saint Augustine

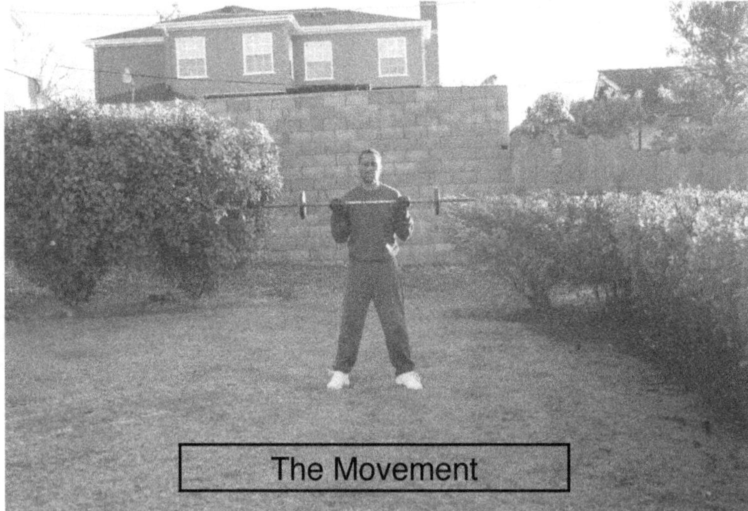

The Movement

The Exercise: With your back straight and your elbows at your sides, lock your legs and hips into a stationary position and slowly curl the barbell up to your shoulders. (Don't throw the weight up by swinging backwards.) Now lower the bar back to the starting point while exhaling.

Workout B - Arms (Biceps)

Standing Dumbbell Curl

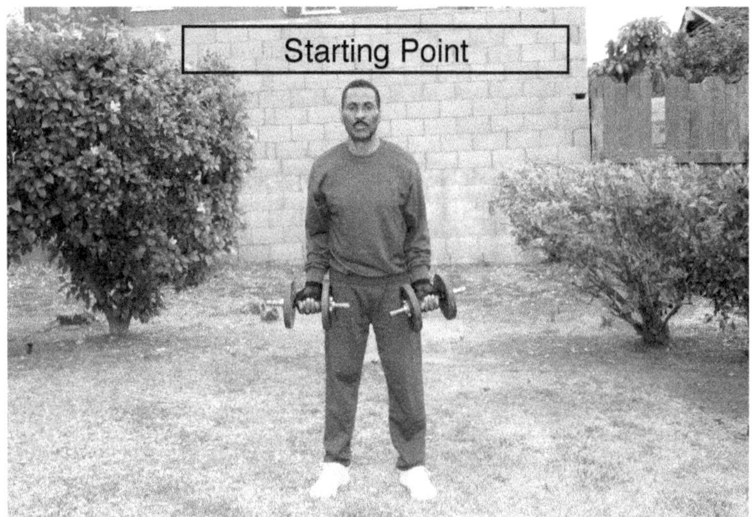

Starting Position: Stand with a dumbbell in each hand. While keeping your elbows at your sides, slowly lift each dumbbell up at the same time while keeping your back straight and avoiding the temptation to throw your shoulders back to aide the movement upwards.

"The present moment is creative, creating with an unheard-of intensity."–Le Corbusier

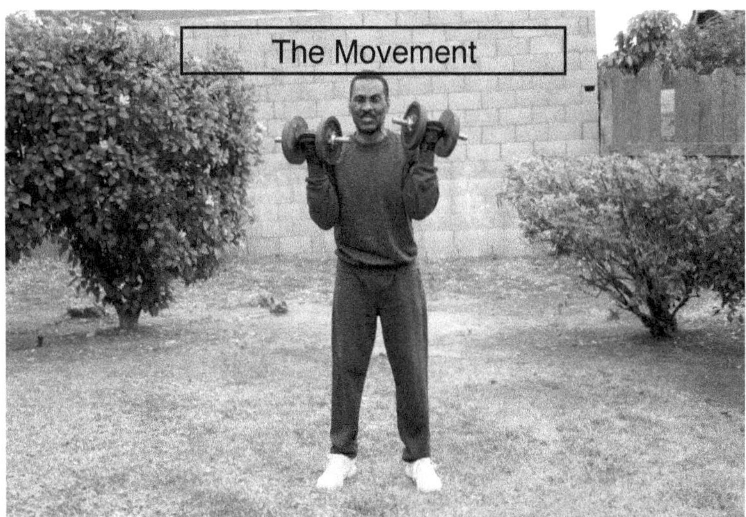

The Exercise: Inhale and curl both dumbbells simultaneously while keeping your palms up throughout the exercise.

Workout B - Arms (Biceps)

Seated Dumbbell Concentration Curl

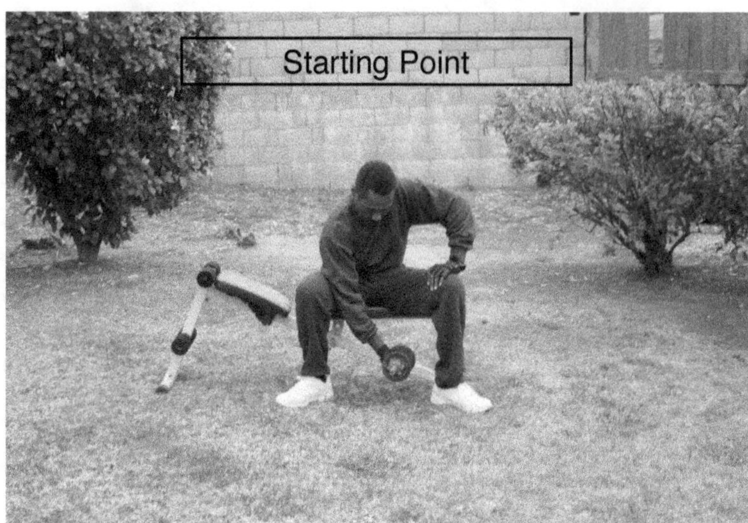

Starting Position: While holding a dumbbell in your right hand at arm's length between your legs, place your left hand on your left thigh to support you, then bend over slightly at the waist. Rest your upper right elbow four inches behind your right knee against your inner thigh.

"Success is going from failure to failure without loss of enthusiasm."–Sir Winston Churchill

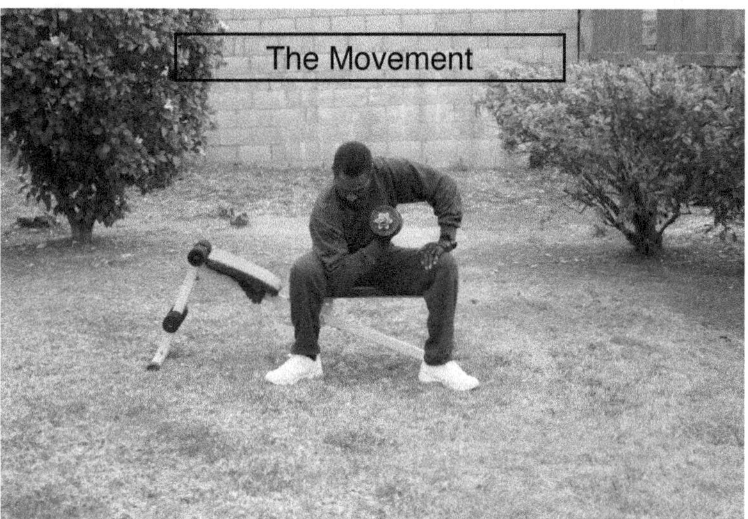

The Exercise: Curl your dumbbell up in an arc-like manner until it almost touches your shoulder. Once at the top, rotate your hand inward to get maximum muscle contraction, then lower it in the same arc pathway. Switch arms and repeat the same way for the other arm.

Workout B - Arms (Biceps)

Seated Dumbbell Alternate Curl

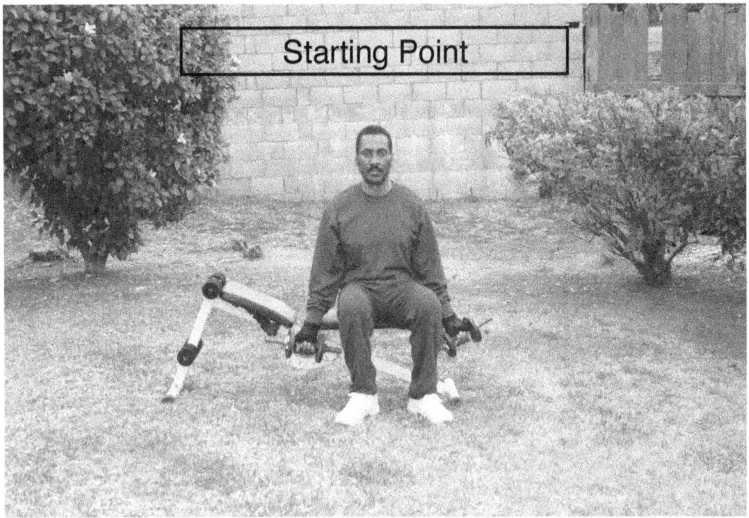

Starting Position: Making sure that your back is straight, head up and feet flat on the floor, sit on a bench with a dumbbell in each hand hanging at arm's length at your sides.

"Happiness is often the result of being too busy to be miserable."–Anonymous

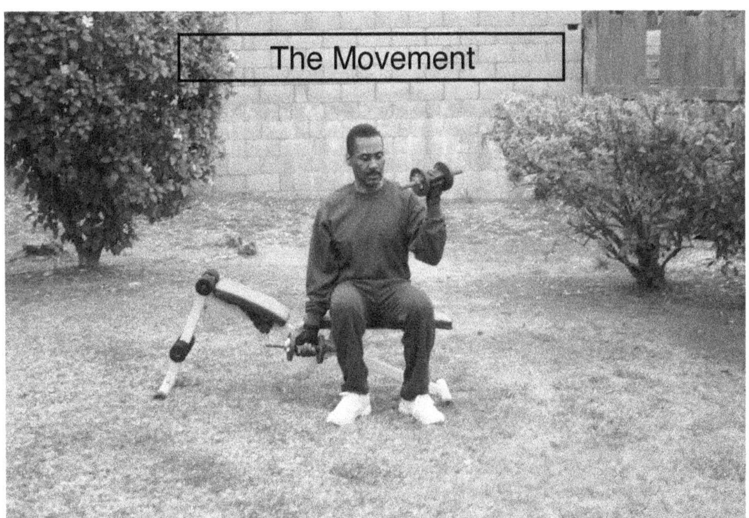

The Exercise: Curling the dumbbells alternately first right then left – left then right. Keep your elbows at your sides and your palms up throughout the movement making sure to raise and lower the weights slowly.

Workout B - Arms (Biceps)

Dumbbell Hammer Curl

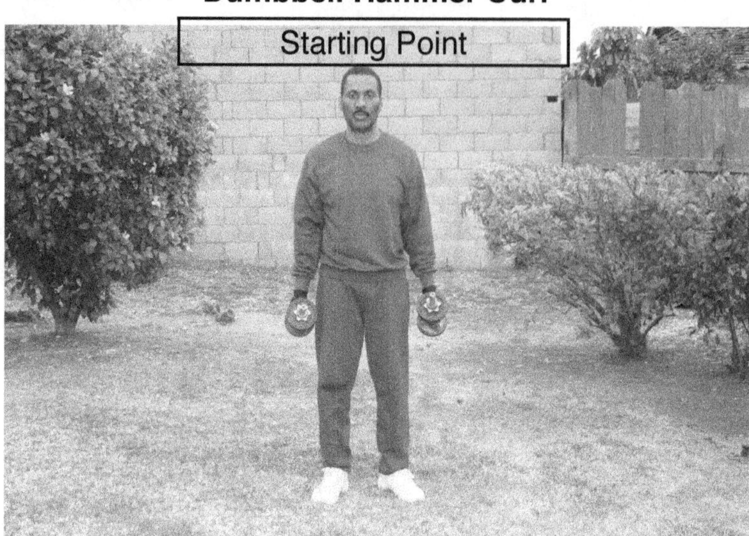

Starting Position: Stand, shoulder-width apart with a dumbbell in each hand, with your arms extended downward at your sides. The key is that the palms must be facing each other.

"The pleasure you get from solving a problem is the purpose and the reward of the problem itself."–Charles Prosper

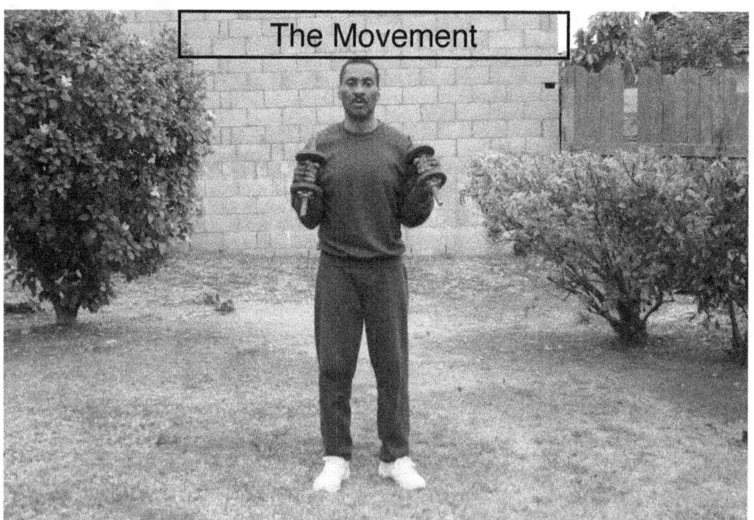

The Exercise: Curl both of your arms upwards to your shoulders. Keep your upper body still by tightening your abs and not leaning too much to the front or to the back. You should actually look as though your are hammering down with the bottom plates.

Workout B - Arms (Forearms)

Seated Barbell Wrist Curl

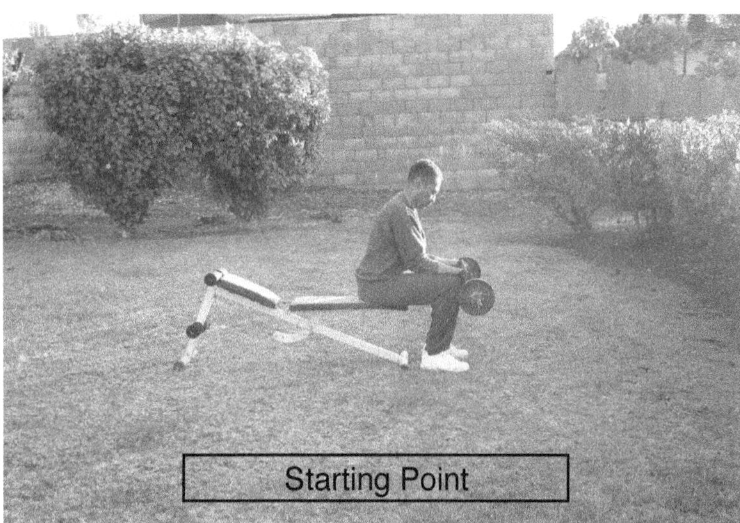

Starting Point

Starting Position: With your foreams resting on thighs and knees (or on the edge of the bench), take an under-handed grip on the barbell with your wrists passively flexed.

"A problem is that you have defined it as so."–Charles Prosper

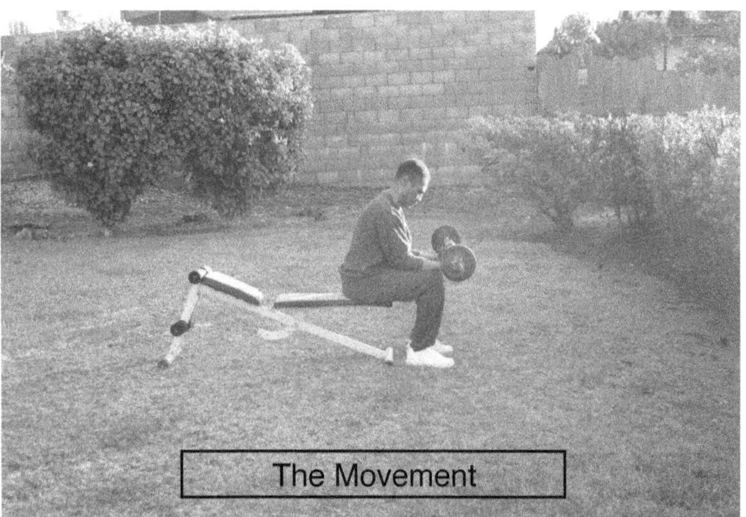

The Movement

The Exercise: Inhale and curl your wrists up and exhale as you complete the movement. This exercise works the large flexor muscles of the forearms.

Workout B - Arms (Forearms)

Seated Barbell Reverse Wrist Curl

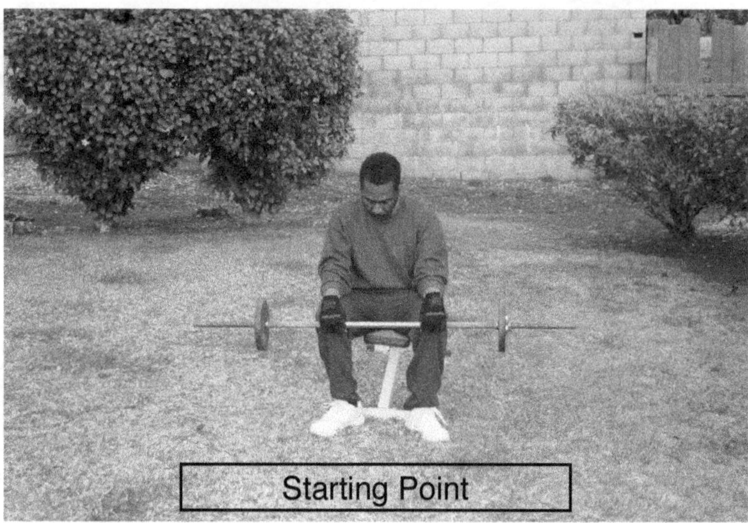

Starting Point

Starting Position: With your foreams resting on thighs and knees (or on the edge of the bench), take an over-handed grip on the barbell with your wrists passively extended downwards.

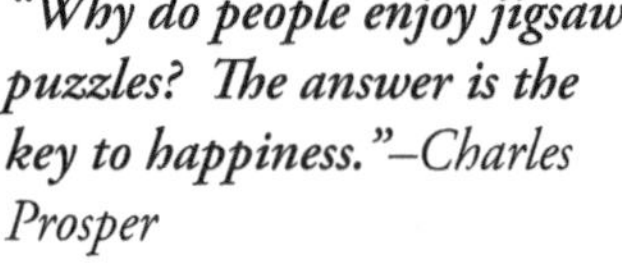

"Why do people enjoy jigsaw puzzles? The answer is the key to happiness."–Charles Prosper

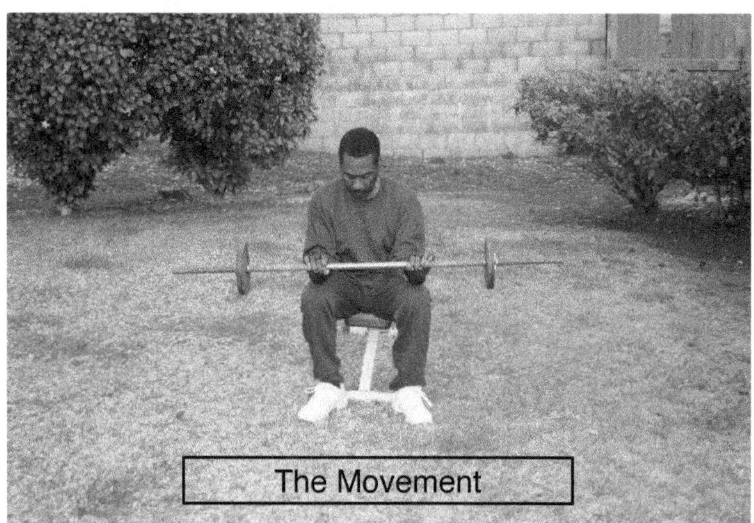

The Movement

The Exercise: With the bar, curl your wrists back towards you. Lower back to the starting movement to begin again for another repetition. This exercise is excellent for developing and strengthening the wrist and finger extensor muscles.

Workout B - Arms (Forearms)

Seated Dumbell Wrist Curl

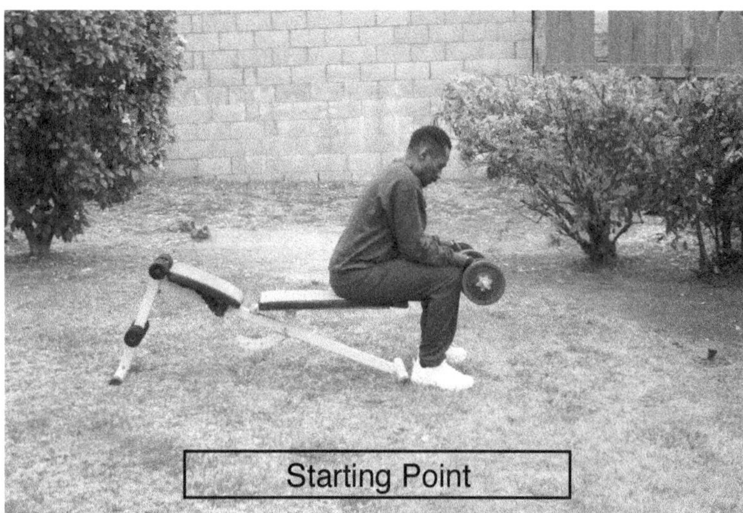

Starting Point

Starting Position: Grab two dumbbells, and with your foreams resting on thighs and knees (or on the edge of the bench), take an under-handed grip on the dumbbells with your wrists passively flexed.

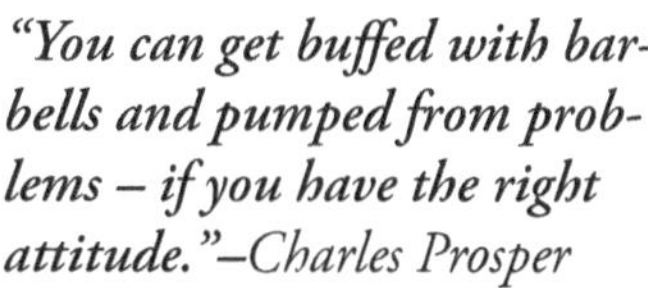

"You can get buffed with barbells and pumped from problems – if you have the right attitude."–Charles Prosper

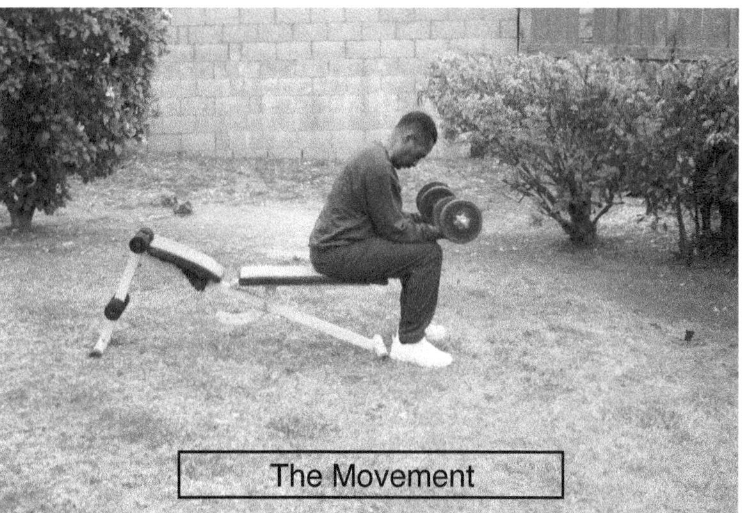

The Movement

The Exercise: Inhale and curl your wrists up and exhale as you complete the movement. This exercise works the large flexor muscles of the forearms even more intensely than with the barbell. A great forearm exercise!

Workout B - Arms (Forearms)

Seated Dumbbell Reverse Wrist Curl

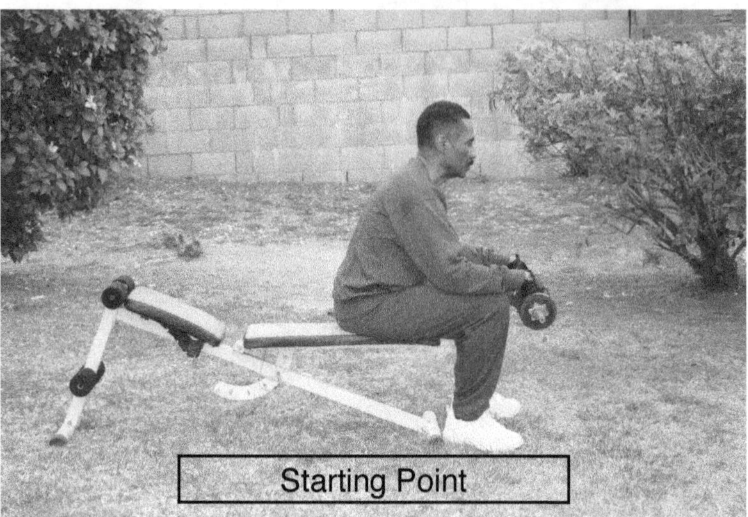

Starting Point

Starting Position: With your foreams resting on thighs and knees (or on the edge of the bench), take an over-handed grip on two dumbbels with your wrists passively extended downwards.

"Fear is faithlessness."–George MacDonald

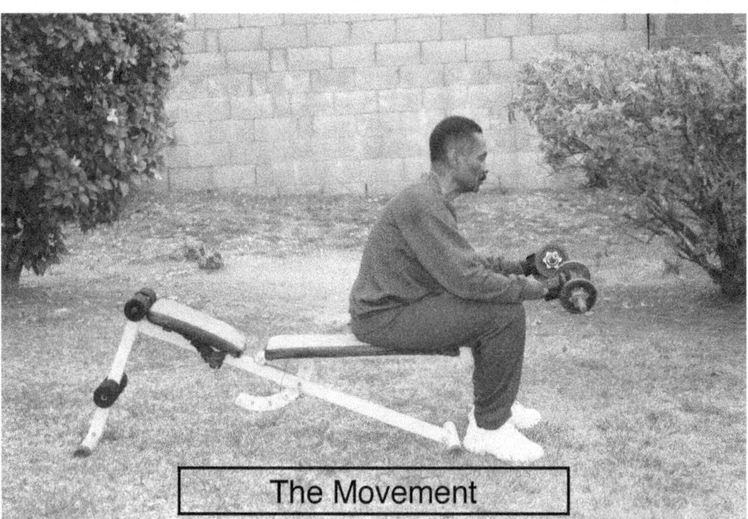

The Movement

The Exercise: With a dumbbell in each hand, curl your wrists back towards you. Lower back to the starting movement to begin again for another repetition. This exercise is excellent for developing and strengthening the wrist and finger extensor muscles.

Workout C - Legs (Quadriceps)

Barbell Squat

Starting Point

Starting Position: Preferably, you should take a barbell off of a squat rack. (Wrap a small towel around the bar to provide comfort at the neck.) Rest the barbell across your upper back with your hands grasping the bar. Keep your head up, back straight, and feet shoulder-width apart.

"No one grows old by living, only by losing interest in living."–Marie Beynon Ray

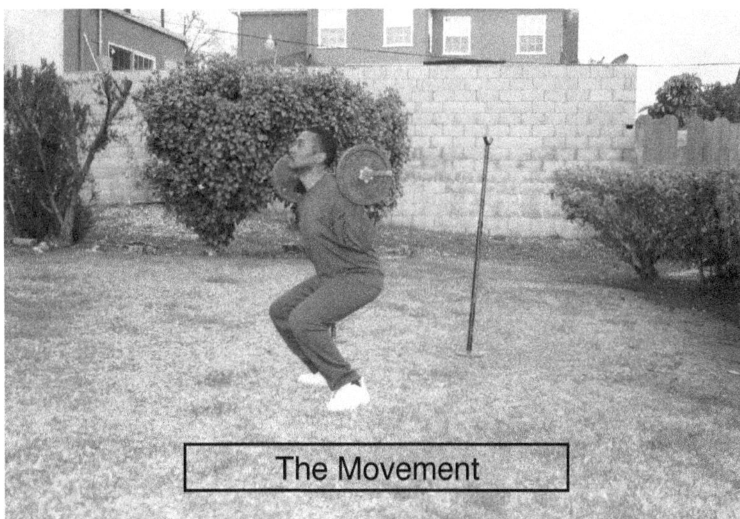

The Movement

The Exercise: Inhale and squat down slowly until your upper thighs are parallel to the floor, then rise carefully back to starting position. (Do not bounce at the bottom as this may injure your knees, and do not lean forward as this will injure your back.)

Workout C - Legs (Quadriceps)

Leg Extensions

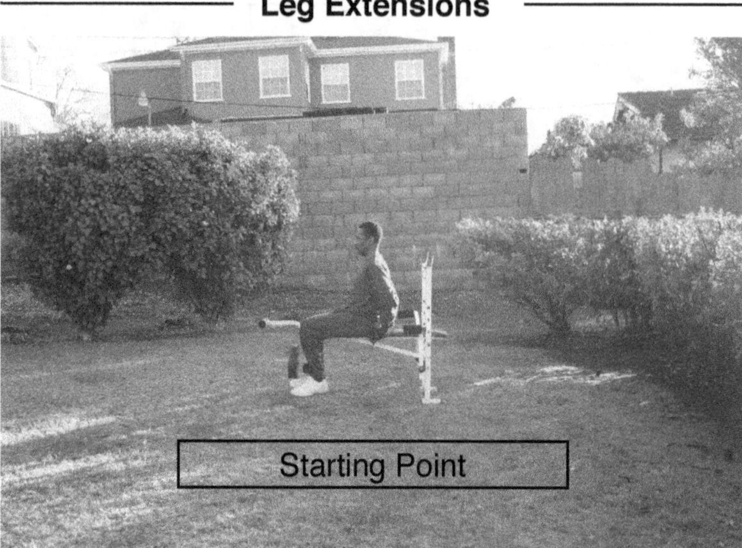

Starting Point

Starting Position: Sit on the edge of your leg extension bench. Hook your feet under the foot pads. Have your knees rest up against the end of the seat. Grab the sides of the bench just below your buttocks, and point your toes straight ahead.

"Success is due less to ability than to zeal."–Charles Buxton

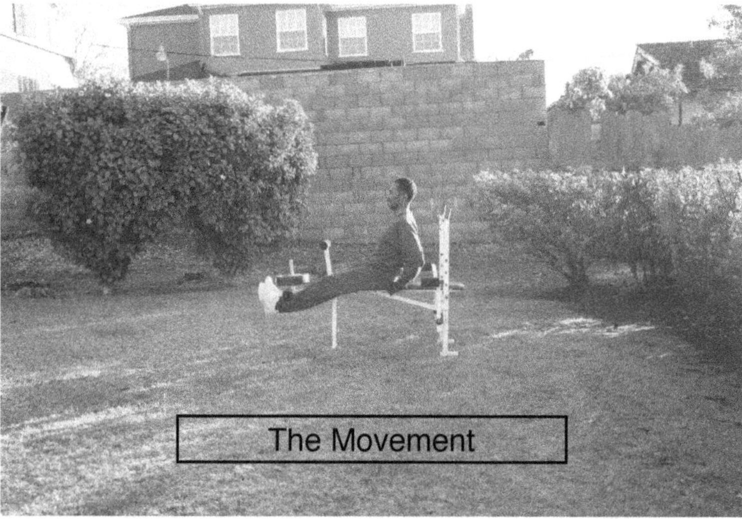

The Movement

The Exercise: While keeping your buttocks on the seat throughout the movement, inhale and raise your legs up until they are extended out. Make sure that you sit up straight throughout the exercise.

Workout C - Legs (Quadriceps)

Forward Dumbbell Lunges

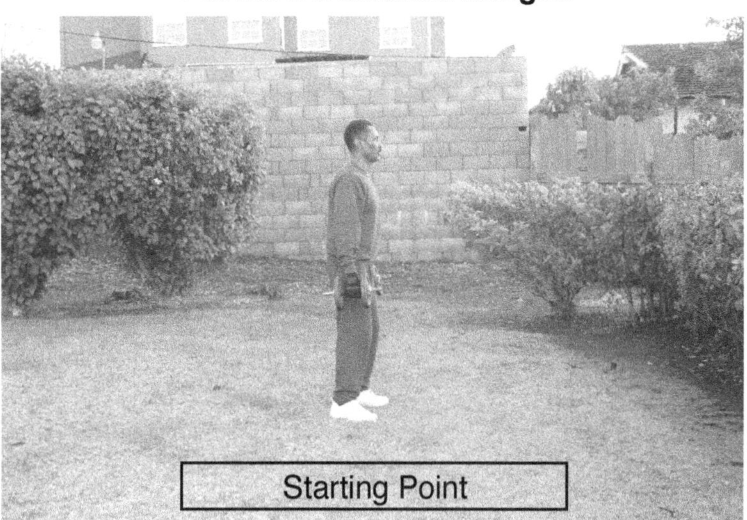

Starting Point

Starting Position: Stand and hold one dumbbell in each hand with your palms facing inward. Keep your head up and your back straight with your feet placed about a foot apart.

"In school, you're taught a lesson and then given a test. In life, you're given a test that teaches you a lesson."–Tom Bodett

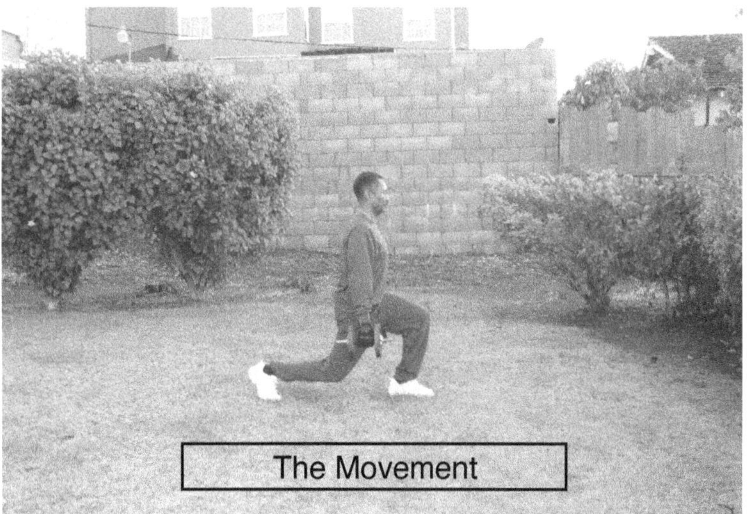

The Movement

The Exercise: Inhale and step forward with your right foot in one smooth movement. Lower your right thigh until it is parallel to the floor. Do not bend your left knee behind you until it is a few inches from the floor. Switch legs. You should feel the stretch in the buttocks and hamstrings.

Workout C - Legs (Quadriceps)

Dumbbell Squats

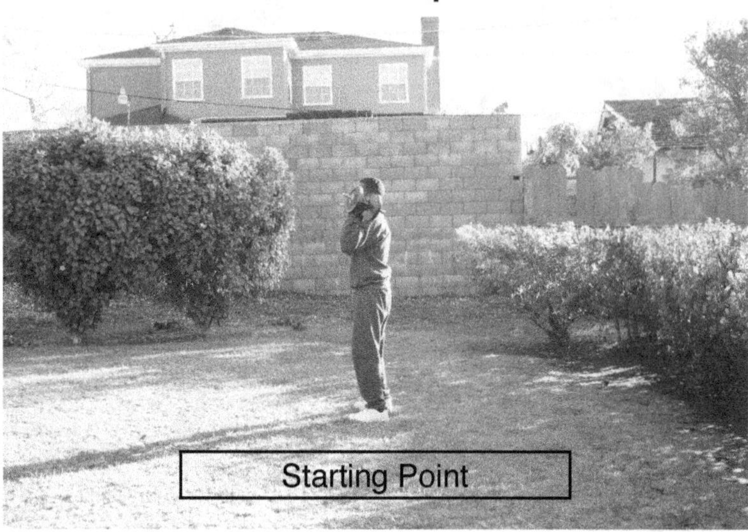

Starting Point

Starting Position: Standing shoulder-width apart, with your palms facing inwards, hold two dumbbells at your sides. For better balance, you may also place a one-inch-thick wooden block or maybe a couple of small dumbbell plates under your heels.

"Passions are the only orators which always persuade."– Francois de La Rochefoucauld

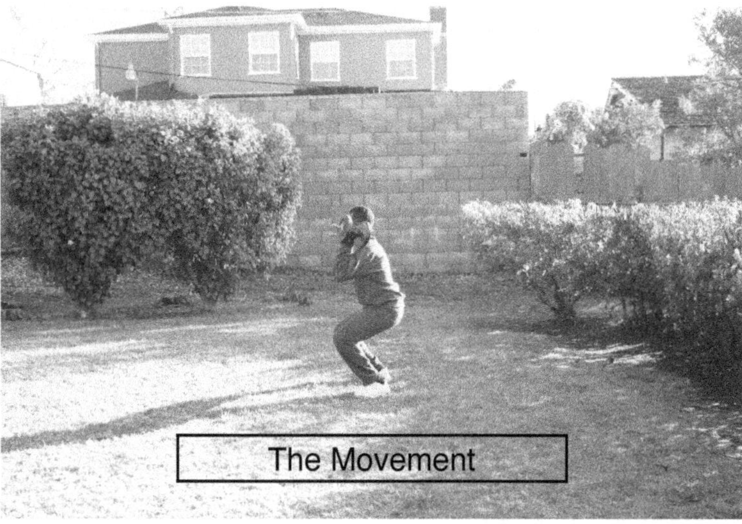

The Movement

The Exercise: Bend your legs at the knees and lower your hips until they are parallel to the floor. You must keep your back straight throughout this movement. Now stand and lift yourself back up to the starting position.

Workout C - Legs (Hamstrings)

Lying Leg Curls

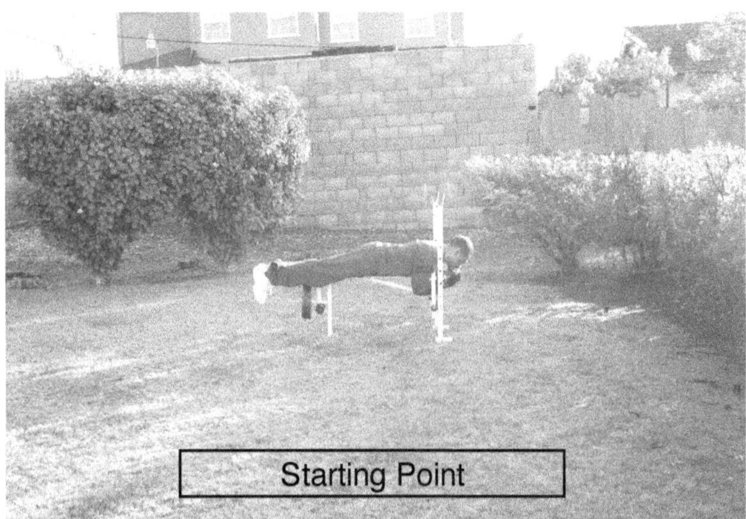

Starting Point

Starting Position: Start by lying face down on your leg curling machine. Make sure the pads are resting on the back of your ankles as your begin to lift.

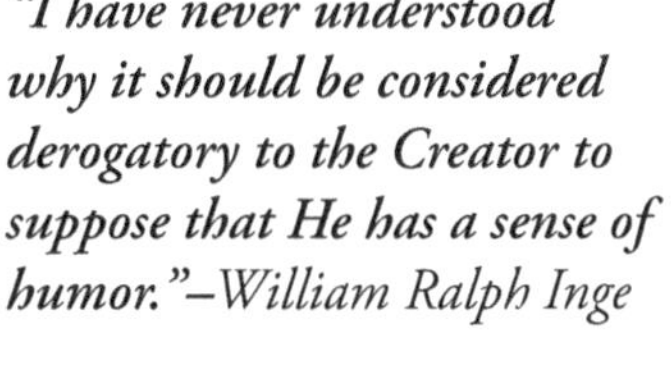

"I have never understood why it should be considered derogatory to the Creator to suppose that He has a sense of humor."–William Ralph Inge

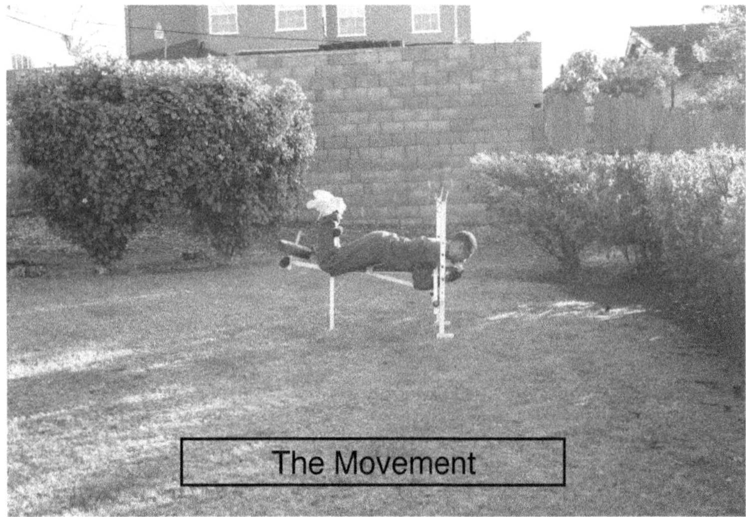

The Movement

The Exercise: As you curl your legs up, you should try to bring your feet as close to your hips as you can. Be sure not to lift your hips up as you curl for this will place unnecessary stress on your lower back.

Workout C - Calves

Seated Barbell Toe Raises

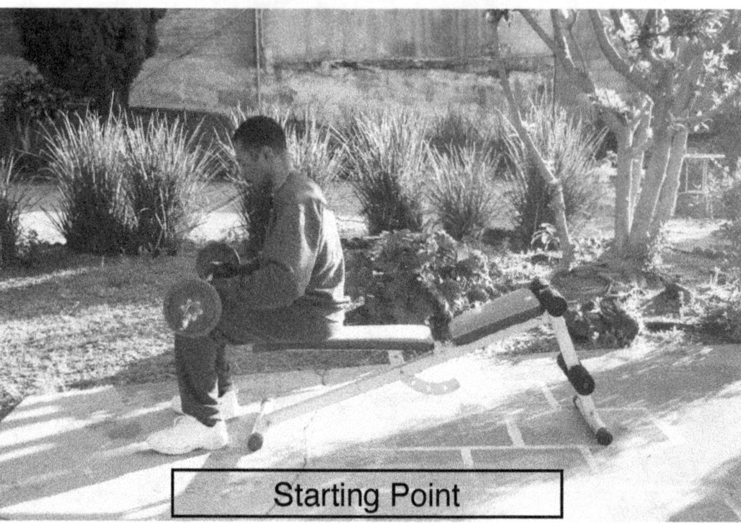

Starting Point

Starting Position: Sit on the edge of a workout bench and place your toes and the balls of your feet on a toe block. Rest the barbell across your lower thighs about three inches behind your knees, holding the bar with your palms down.

"Curse the problem, and see your suffering. Bless the problem, and see your solution."–Charles Prosper

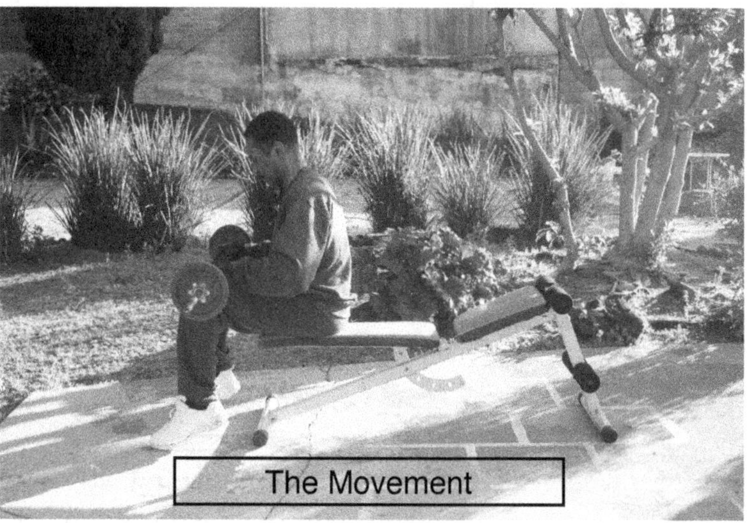

The Movement

The Exercise: Raise your toes up as high as you can while keeping your back straight and your head up. Hold the top position for two seconds then lower back to the starting position. With seated toe raises, you can do more reps than normal. Shoot for 50 or until it burns.

Workout C - Calves

Angled Barbell Calf Raises

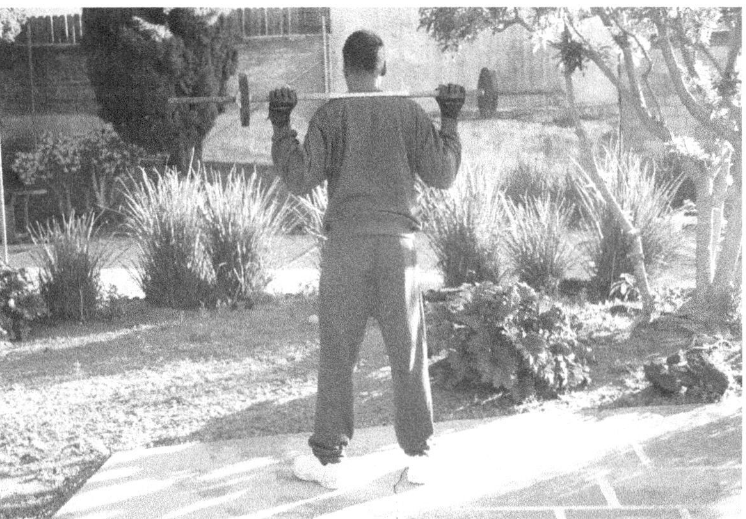

Starting Position: Place a barbell across your upper back while firmly gripping the bar. Keep your head up, your back straight and your feet shoulder-width apart. Now turn your toes outwards so that your feet form a 45° angle.

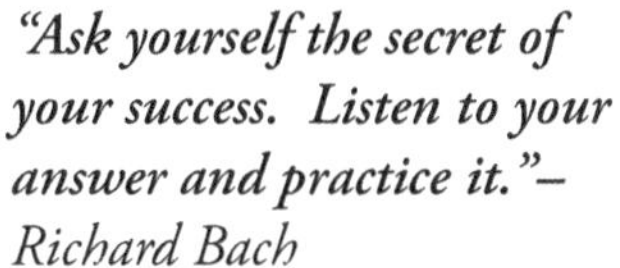

"Ask yourself the secret of your success. Listen to your answer and practice it."– Richard Bach

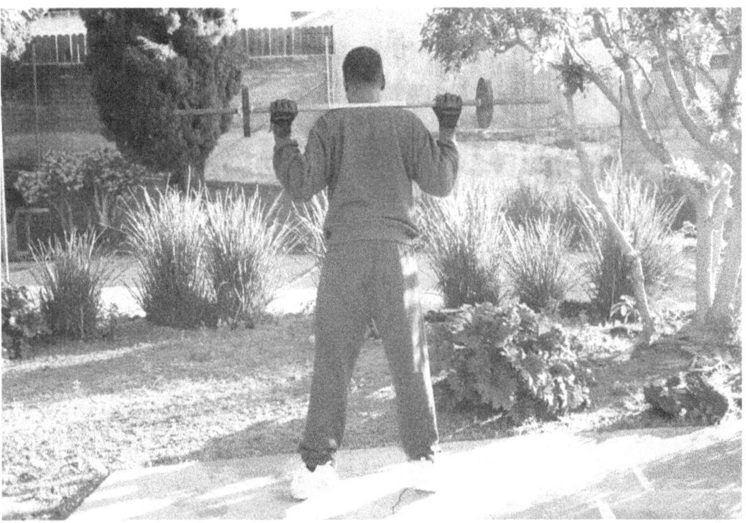

The Exercise: While keeping your legs straight, raise up on your toes as high as you can. Hold the top position for a count of one then slowly lower your feet back down to the starting position.

Workout C - Calves

One-Legged Calf Raises

Starting Point

Starting Position: Stand on the ball of your right foot on a sturdy block with a dumbbell in your left hand, and with your right hand, hold on to something to keep your balance. Hook your left foot around your right calf. Now lift your right foot up as high as you can.

"Every tomorrow has two handles. We can take hold of it with the handle of anxiety or the handle of faith."– Henry Ward Beecher

The Movement

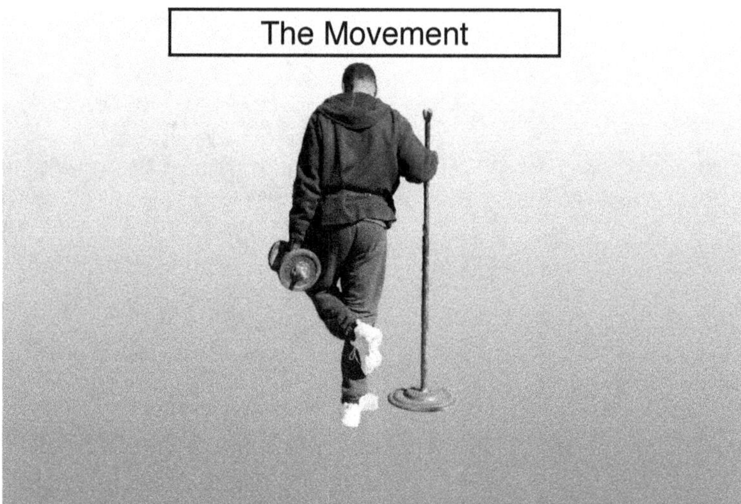

The Exercise: Lower your right heel as far as you can, stretching the calf muscle as much as possible. Now press up high on your toes to contract the muscle. Make sure that you put the weight on the ball of your foot. Switch to the other leg and repeat. 20+ reps are good.

Workout C - Calves

Angled Dumbbell Calf Raises

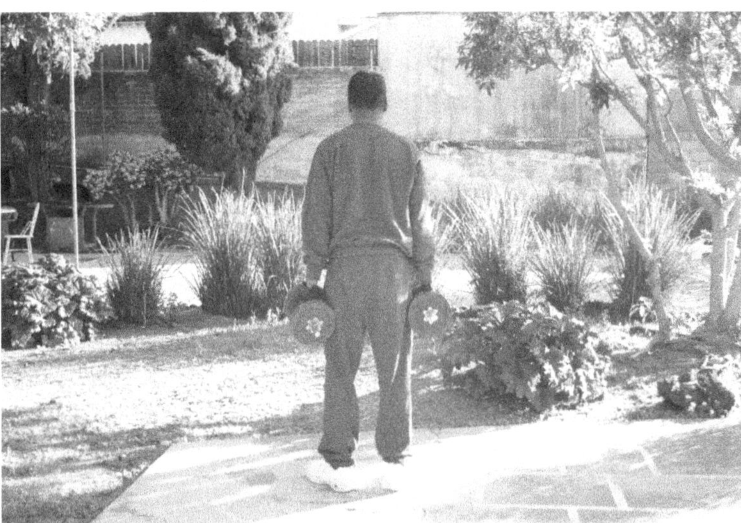

Starting Position: Hold a dumbbell in each hand. Keep your head up, your back straight and your feet shoulder-width apart. Now turn your toes outwards so that your feet form a 45° angle.

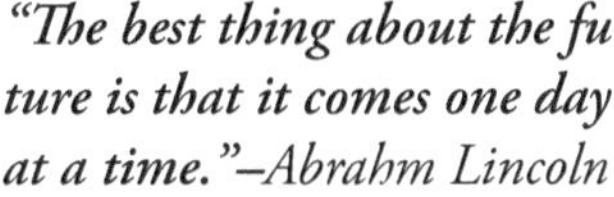

"The best thing about the future is that it comes one day at a time."–Abrahm Lincoln

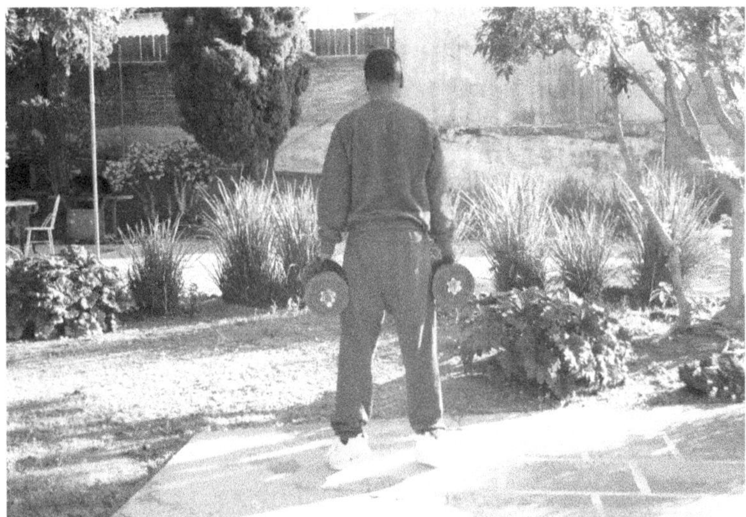

The Exercise: While keeping your legs straight, raise up on your toes as high as you can. Hold the top position for a count of one then slowly lower your feet back down to the starting position.

Workout C - Abs

Bench Ab Crunches

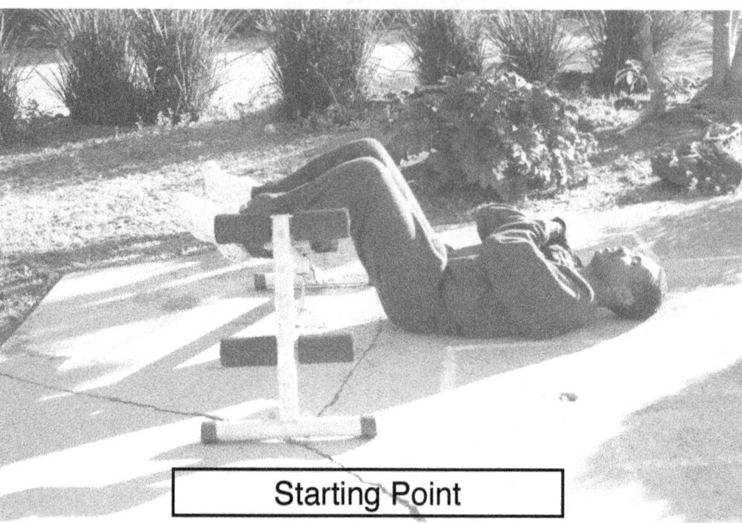

Starting Point

Starting Position: Lie on the floor and cross your arms across your chest. Keeping your knees together, place your lower legs over a bench having your legs form a 90° angle on the floor.

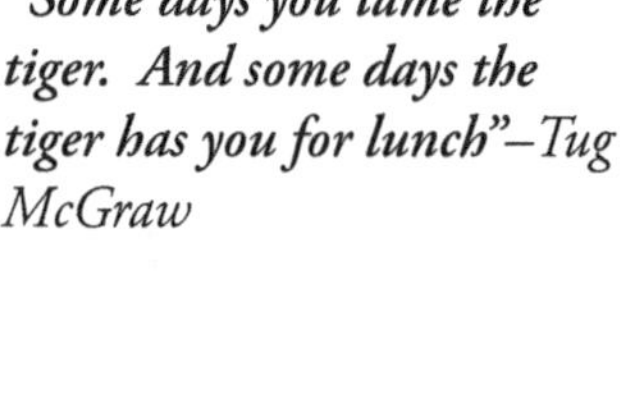

"Some days you tame the tiger. And some days the tiger has you for lunch"–Tug McGraw

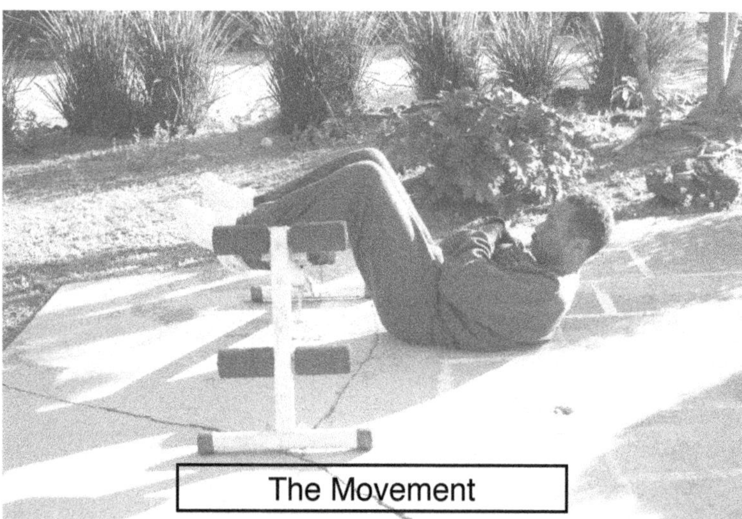

The Movement

The Exercise: Roll your breastbone (sternum) up towards your pelvis while keeping your hips and knees locked into place. You are to hold the top position while squeezing your abs once before going back down to the starting position.

Workout C - Abs

Doorway Hanging Leg Raises

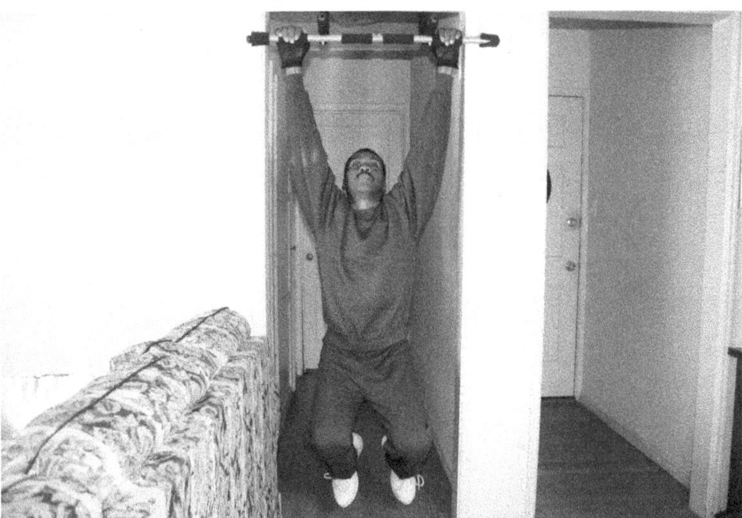

"Pain is never permanent."– Saint Teresa of Avila

Starting Position: Grab a chinning bar with your palms facing outwards. Hang from the bar keeping your arms straight throughout the exercise. The focus is on your pelvis which is to roll forward towards the bar.

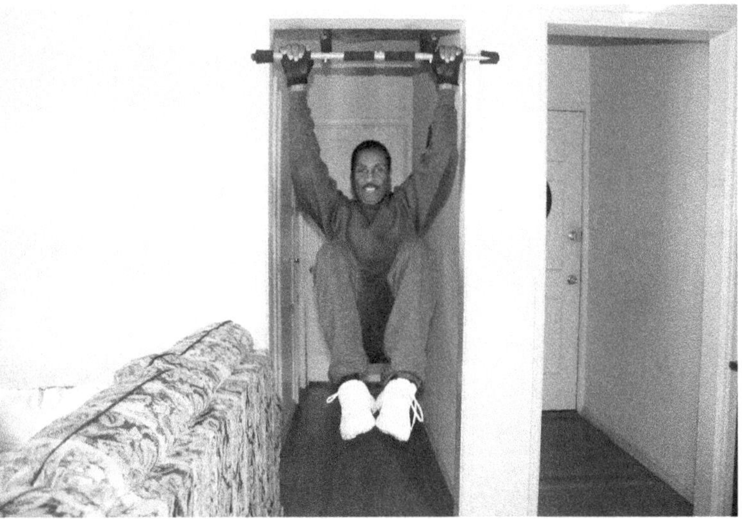

The Exercise: While hanging with your knees bent, raise them until they are parallel to the floor, and exhale. Instead of arching your back, just keep it a little rounded. Now slowly lower your legs back to the starting position and repeat for the desired number of reps.

Workout C - Abs

Lying Leg Raises

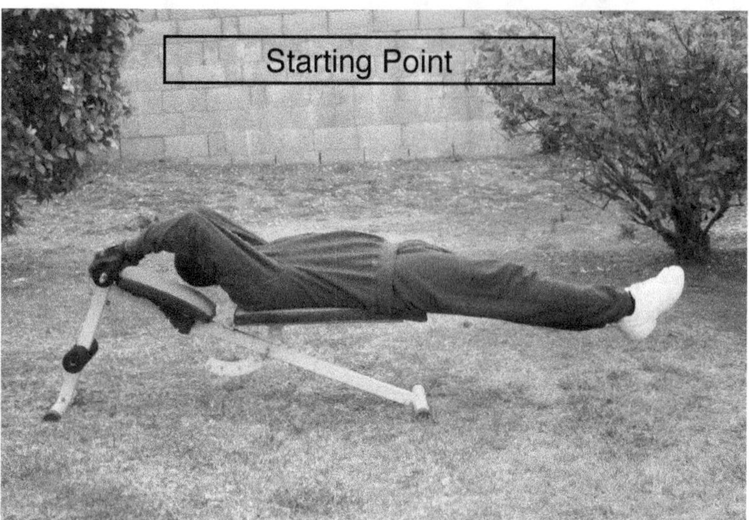

Starting Position: Lie flat on a bench so that your buttocks are on the end. Now grab your hands above your head and hold on to the top of the bench. Point your toes and raise your legs until they are parallel to the floor and half your body is a straight line off the edge of the bench.

"Patience is a bitter plant, but it has sweet fruit."– German Proverb

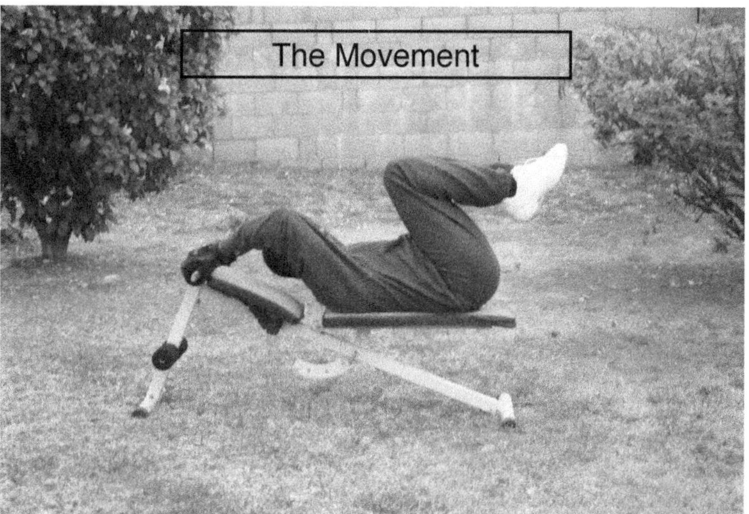

The Exercise: As you inhale, bend your knees and draw your upper thighs into your midsection region while simultaneously raising your head and shoulders to meet your thighs. Slightly curve your back and tilt your pelvis, then slowly lower back down to the straight-line starting position.

Workout C - Abs

Declined Sit-Ups

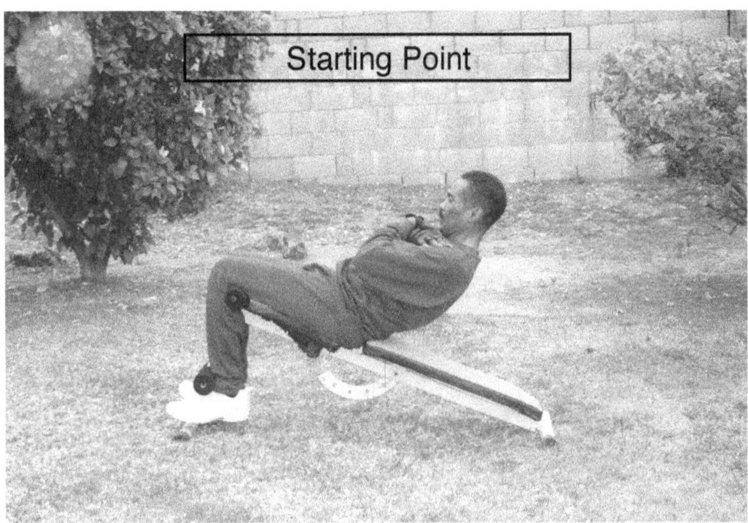

Starting Position: Lie down on a declined bench, and your feet under the pads. Sit up as high as you can. Now place your hands across your chest. Do not lock your fingers behind your head for this causes you to pull your neck down putting bad stress on your spine.

"Genius is nothing but a greater aptitude for patience."–Benjamin Franklin

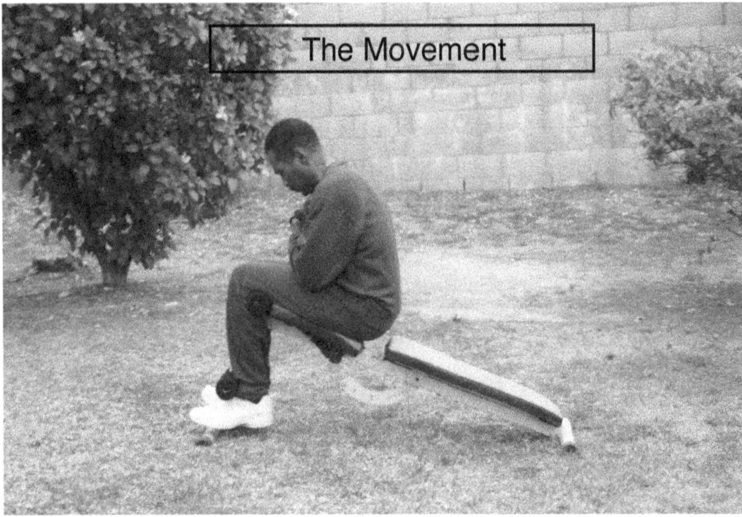

The Exercise: While starting from the upper position, begin by contracting your abs, and go back only one foot. Do not go back all of the way as this will place harmful stress on your back. As you become stronger than 12 reps, do it with a 10 lb. plate held against your sternum.

A Little Note on Working The Deltoid (Shoulders)

The deltoid muscle is derived from the etymological root "delta" which in the case of the deltoid muscle is shaped like an upside-down triangle (or Dorito® chip). I point this out to say that when you are selecting a variety of new shoulder-muscle exercises to do, keep in mind that your deltoid (shoulder) muscle has three heads:

- the frontal head
- the lateral head
- the rear head

Understanding this, you will alternately select exercises, that at some point, will exercise each of these three heads. This allows you to develop an esthetically pleasing deltoid muscle with a balanced development on all three sides.

There *are* specific shoulder exercises that emphasize each of the three heads respectively. For example the:

"We do not remember days, we remember moments."– *Cesare Pavese*

- standing barbell press develops the *frontal heads*
- lateral dumbbell raises develops the *lateral heads*
- bent-over dumbbell lateral raises develop the *rear heads*

Notice All of The Exercises Are Shown With Free Weights

Did you notice something curious about the selection of exercises that I gave you? If you did, you would have noticed that they practically all were with free weights, that is, barbells and dumbbells. (The only minor exception, if you want to consider it as such, are the leg curls and the leg extension exercises which require this standard attachment that is found on most home-gym workout benches.)

Sure, if you are a member of a professional gym, you will indeed be in Shangri-la, in that you will have a plethora of workout machine possibilities to choose from, and that is fine if that is the case, but the point that I am trying to make is that there is NO excuse for you not to start. I developed the body that I have over the last 4 years, exclusively by using the simple barbell, bench and dumbbell equipment that I purchased for my home gym which I use regularly and religiously in the open air of my garden that is in the back of my house. I think that the total I have invested in my equipment has not been more than $350.00.

So, what's your excuse for not starting? Are you waiting for the perfect gym with the snazziest equipment? Do you believe that you need a personal trainer barking commands for you to lift this and squat that? Look, don't get me wrong. I have had more than one personal trainer in my life. I have to admit that I learned something from each trainer I've had, and I've made excellent gains from each, but if for some reason a gym membership or a personal trainer is not practical for you at the present time, don't wait for the perfect situation. Do what you can with where you are and with whom you are. Just *do* it. And do it now!

Remember, ordinary things consistently done bring extraordinary results.

"If you do not ask yourself what it is you know, you will go on listening to others and change will not come because you will not hear your own truth." *–Saint Bartholomew*

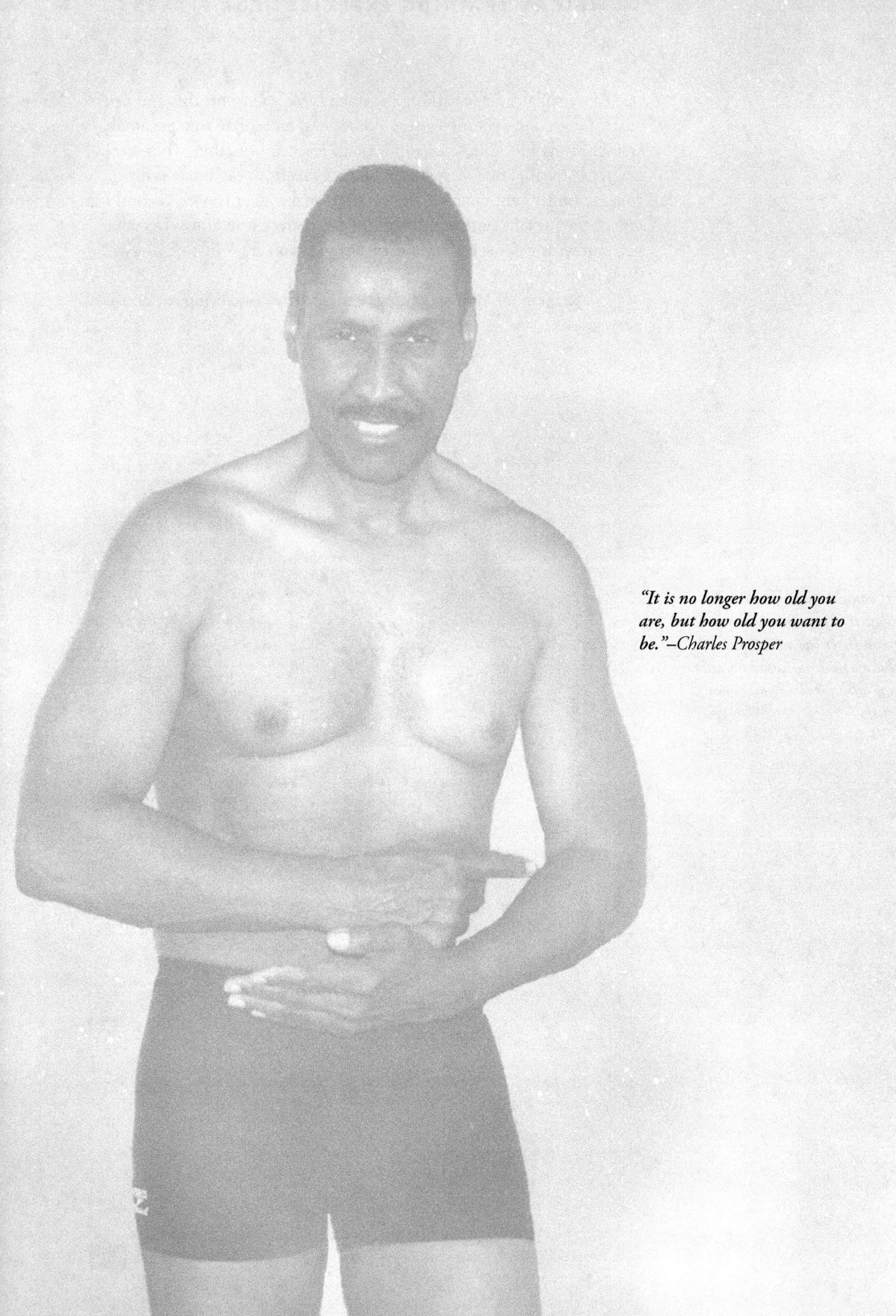

"It is no longer how old you are, but how old you want to be."–Charles Prosper

CHAPTER 11

Gym Membership or Home Gym – The Benefits of Both

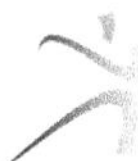

Okay, now you've made your decision that you are ready to start and that you are fired up and committed to stay with it until you reach your goal. Now comes the decision of where to train. Should you go for the monthly gym membership, or should you just go over to Big 5® sporting goods store and purchase an inexpensive set of barbells, dumbbells and a workout bench? Actually, you can do either and become successful at achieving your ultimate health and fitness goals.

To help you sort out the pros and the cons of each, let us take a positive look at the respective benefits of each, and the drawbacks of both will become obvious in order for you to make an informed decision according to your situation and to your needs.

"Happiness is action."–David Thomas

We will first take a look at the advantages of a gym membership. Then we will examine the advantages of purchasing a home gym.

The 4 Advantages of Gym Membership

When it comes to gym membership, I know that some people are almost evangelical in their zeal in support of this route. Belonging to a gym is great if you can afford it and if it is conveniently located. But enough of my skimming the surface, what are the 4 advantages of gym membership?

- **A Wide Variety of Exercise Equipment**
- **Availability of Personal Trainers**
- **A Total Workout Ambience**
- **Opportunity to Meet Like-Minded Members**

Advantage #1 *(Gym Membership)* – A Wide Variety of Equipment

One thing is for sure, you will never get bored by not having enough variety of exercise possibilities. In a professional gym, there is a plethora of barbells, dumbbells, calf machines, lat machines, thigh machines, inclined benches, declined benches, stationary bicycles, moving treadmills and more. There is even, usually, 360° of mirrors to admire yourself as you progress more and more. Once you become an aficionado of the health and fitness magazines, and when you want to try out a new exercise that you may read about, you are almost certain to find the exercise equipment in your gym.

Advantage #2 *(Gym Membership)* – Availability of Personal Trainers

Nothing can get you off to a better start – *and* to keep you on track better than a good personal trainer. And I do emphasize *good* here. Should you choose a mediocre trainer, at best, you are better on your own. Choosing a reputable and qualified personal trainer, with your motivation and your willingness to follow through and your commitment to succeed, I can see that your success is *guaranteed.*

Advantage #3 *(Gym Membership)* – A Total Workout Ambience

Once you are submerged in the total gym environment, you virtually do not have time to think of anything else. There are no outside-world distractions to take you away from what you are doing. (Unless you carry a cell phone around with you when you workout - *Duh!)* You are surrounded in a sea of successfully-built bodies which can also serve to keep you motivated as well.

Advantage #4 *(Gym Membership)* – Meeting Like-Minded Members

"Act as if it were impossible to fail."–Dorothea Brande

If you are a gregarious type, as most of us are to some degree, you can enjoy meeting like-minded gym members who maybe once started where you are now, and have achieved great strides. This is the purpose of the "club" part in Health Club. Like-minded people, when they gather and talk mutually about their passion, tend to inspire, fire up and motivate each other even more.

The 6 Advantages of Owning A Home Gym

If you pick up any typical health and fitness magazine that emphasizes muscularity and body sculpture, you will notice that very little credence is given to the home gym. It is as though a home gym were not an equally viable alternative – which in my 5-year experience has shown to be just as effective as a professional gym, as long as you are committed and are consistent. Here are the 6 advantages of owning a home gym:

- **Your Home Gym Is Available 24/7**
- **You Are Free of Monthly Gym Fees**
- **You Don't Have to Leave Home and Drive Out**
- **You Don't Have to Worry About Athlete's Foot**
- **You Never Have to Wait to Use Exercise Equipment**
- **It's Never Crowded**

Advantage #1 *(Home Gym)* – It Is Available 24/7

With a home gym, you do not have to adapt yourself to the hours of the gym. If you want to exercise at 3:00 a.m. – you can. If you want to exercise at 11:00 p.m. – you can. Sundays. Holidays. It doesn't matter. Your home gym is always there waiting and ready to serve you by whatever schedule you designate.

Advantage #2 *(Home Gym)* – No Monthly Fees

Once you pay for a piece of equipment, you're done. No more money out of your pocket. In the short run, paying monthly gym fees may not be significant in the first few months, but over the course of 1, 2 or 3 years of monthly gym membership, you could have purchased yourself a mighty snazzy home gym.

Advantage #3 *(Home Gym)* – No Need to Leave Home and Drive Out

Let's say that you have to be to work at 7:40 a.m., and in addition to that you have to get your daughter up, fix breakfast and have her ready for school. (I am sort of describing my own situation.) Well, if you have to begin your workout at 4:00 a.m., you are out of luck for most membership gyms that open up at 5:00 a.m. and 6:00 a.m. And remember, you still have to count in your drive time (and finding parking if it happens to be after work hours when everything is very busy).

"If you would be powerful, pretend to be powerful." *– Horne Tooke*

Advantage #4 *(Home Gym)* – No Need To Worry About Athlete's Foot

Something that very few gym owners like to mention or talk about is how easy it is for you to get athlete's foot by bathing in public gym bathrooms. (And yes, you sometimes get it even when you wear those rubber beach sandals.) Once that grungy fungus gets between your toes, you can expect a burning itch-fest for many days or weeks to come.

Advantage #5 *(Home Gym)* – No Need To Wait to Use Equipment

If it is a busy time of the day, like at about 5:00 to 6:00 p.m. when everyone is getting off from work to go to the gym, you can expect that there are going to be a lot of people wanting to use the choice pieces of equipment. Sometimes you will get a self-centered and inconsiderate person who will, say, literally hog the pec deck or the calf-raising machine. Sure you can get into an argument with how they are taking too long, but who wants the hassle?

Advantage #6 *(Home Gym)* – It's Never Crowded

Alluding to advantage #5 of the home gym, again is the simple fact that because it is your personal gym, you need not share it with the public. In short, is it never crowded on your workout floor. If you are one who likes to workout alone in the peace and quiet of your home asylum, a home gym might be just the choice for you.

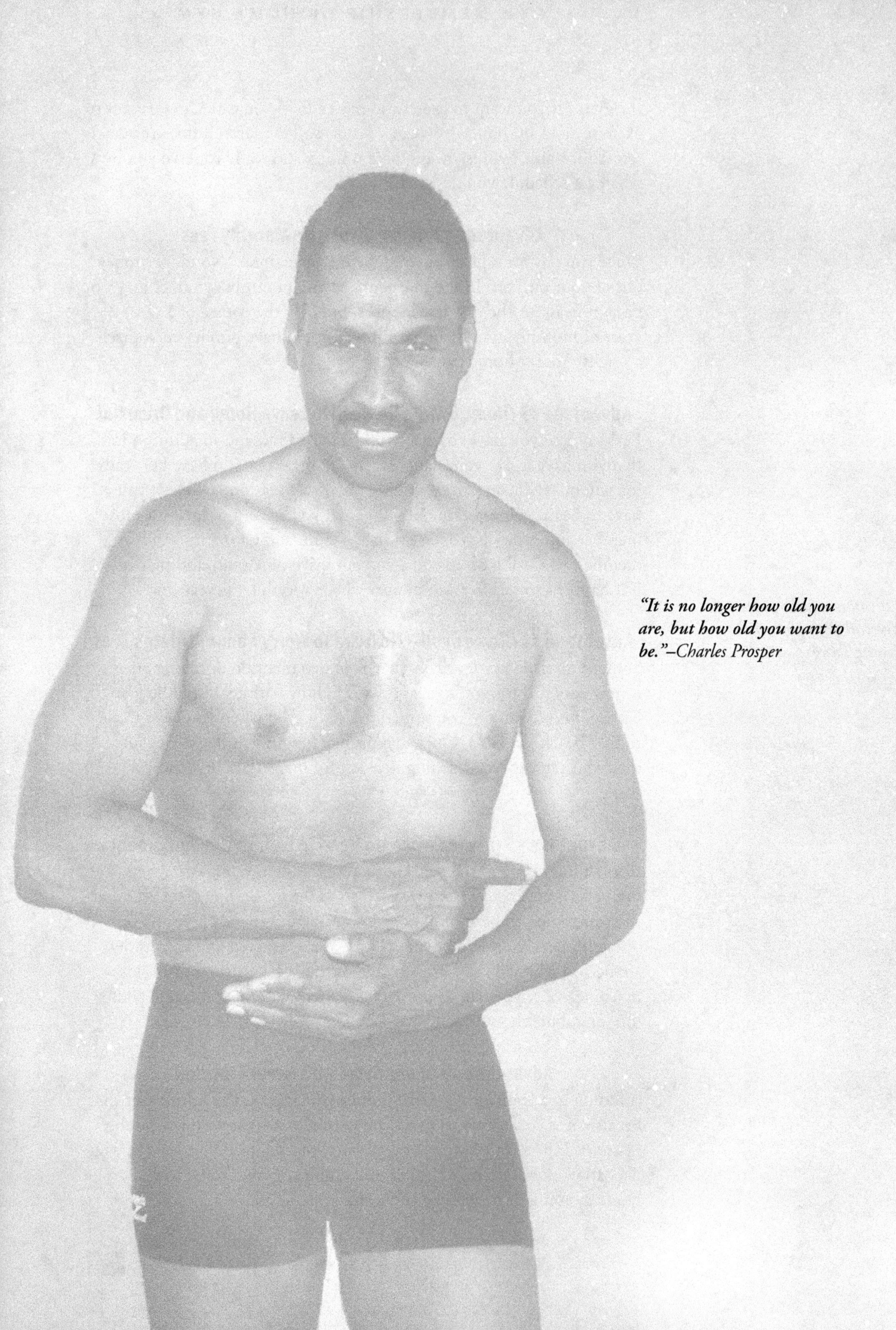

"It is no longer how old you are, but how old you want to be."–Charles Prosper

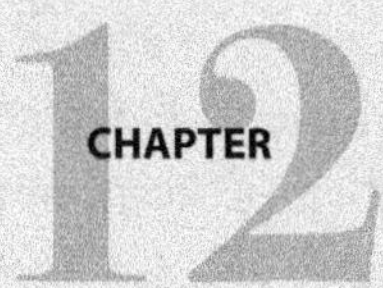

My Youth-Enhancing Herbal Secrets

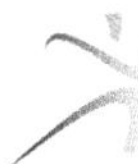

Okay, I am going to indulge myself a bit in order to swing into the explanation of this chapter. People ask me all of the time, how do I manage to look so young! I hardly have a wrinkle on my face and my eyes and skin glow and sparkle with radiant health. I need to slow down a little with my self-adulation before you start to gag. All this is to say that I have what I believe are long-known herbal secrets that can do incredible things to maintain your face, eyes and skin healthy and radiant. It is just a matter of knowing what they are and then to follow through with the willingness to use them on a daily and regular basis. Remember my favorite saying, "Ordinary things *consistently* done produce extraordinary results." Now, I offer to you my herbal youth remedies that, used in conjunction with your clean eating, weight resistance exercise, aerobic activity and your vitamins, virtually cannot fail.

"God speaks to all individuals through what happens to them moment by moment."– J.P. DeCaussade

The Fantastic Four of Herbal Secrets

I want to keep things very simple and easy to remember. There are four additions to your regimen that I strongly recommend. These four powerful herbal nutrients are:

- **Flaxseed Oil**
- **Ginseng Extract**
- **Wheat Bran (Unprocessed)**
- **ProGreens by Nutricology®**

The interesting thing about them is that they all, with the exception of the ProGreens® product, have been known for centuries. Many times, individually and selectively, an herbal nutrient will have one effect– but – when you synthesize them by having them work together, a whole new effect and product results. This is why I recommend for you to use all four of these nutrients, and scientifically just see what happens. You will be amazed with the results. Now, let's look closer at each.

Flaxseed Oil

Flaxseed oil, (also known as Linseed oil) that comes from a blue flowering plant is grown on the Western Canadian Prairies. Flaxseed oil contains B vitamins, lecithin, zinc, potassium, fiber, protein, magnesium, omega-3, omega-6 and omega-9 essential fatty acids – *with none of the horrible fishy aftertaste of omega-3 fatty acids obtained from fish oil capsules.*

The Benefits of Flaxseed Oil

- the Omega-3 fatty acids helps lower cholesterol
- helps maintain beautiful hair, skin and nails
- works as an intestinal bowel lubricant aiding elimination
- can improve eyesight and the perception of colors
- increases your metabolism thus helping to burn fat
- can lower high blood pressure from hypertension
- can help in the treatment of depression
- *and much, much, more...*

"Every morning I spend fifteen minutes filling my mind full of God, and so there's no room for worry ."–Howard Chandler Christy

There are many brands and a couple of ways that you can take flaxseed oil: as liquid with a tablespoon or as gelatin capsules. I highly recommend the brand Spectrum Essentials® and their Organic Flaxseed Oil, Omega-3 (Original Flavor) as a liquid. I have found, out of all of the various brands of liquid flaxseed oil, that the flavor of Spectrum Essentials® is absolutely delightful. You can take a tablespoon of it, and I guarantee you will have absolutely no aftertaste. I like putting a couple of tablespoons of flaxseed oil on a fresh green garden salad with a little lemon and salt. Yummy! You don't need that much as a daily dose. If you take just two tablespoons a day, you have taken care of all of the good fats that your body needs for that day.

One other thing, when you look on the Supplement Facts of the bottle label, you will notice that it says, "Calories 120 per tablespoon serving". You will also notice that it says, "Calories from fat 120". In the case of good fats like flaxseed oil, this is a good thing, that the content is 100% fat. Remember, in this case, we are talking about 100% *good* fat! Oh, yes, and flaxseed oil not only has Omega-3, but Omega-6 and Omega-9 healthy fatty acids as well.

Ginseng

Ginseng is an incredibly beneficial plant which has been used by the Chinese for thousands of years. The herbal qualities of ginseng is taken from the root when looked at it creatively, many times has the form and shape of a man with an apparent head shoulders and arms. Ginseng is a plant that the Native American Indians used for centuries as well. The botanical name for Ginseng is also Panax Ginseng. The word Panax is a derivative of the Greek root, meaning "all healing".

The Benefits of Ginseng

- helps to lower cholesterol
- increases physical endurance by holding oxygen longer
- improves the immune system
- slows down the aging process
- improves the body's metabolic fat-burning rate
- aides sleep by regulating sleep cycles
- reduces the effects of stress
- helps to alleviate rheumatism
- believed to help improve sexual libido
- helps to alleviate cough
- helps to treat diabetes by restoring blood sugar levels
- improves mental ability
- improves memory loss from Alzheimer's Disease
- helps to regulate the female body systems

"God is no enemy to you. He asks no more than He hear you call Him "Friend."–A *Course in Miracles*

Ginseng is abundantly found in China, Korea and North America. The root can be boiled in hot water to make a tea, but my favorite way to take ginseng is by drinking the small liquid vial extracts or it can be taken as capsules. I take ginseng first thing in the morning on an empty stomach for better absorption. Great before jogging and weight resistance exercise.

Wheat Bran (Unprocessed)

When you eat bread products made with white bleached processed flour, you are essentially eating bread products that have been stripped of some of the most important parts – like the bran. I recommend that you get an unprocessed wheat bran.

The Benefits of Wheat Bran (Unprocessed)

- helps to keep your digestive system working properly
- may reduce the risk of colon cancer
- helps eliminate accumulated toxins from the colon
- high in B-vitamins
- provides high fiber content and promotes regularity

One of the best unprocessed wheat brans on the market is Millers Bran of Hodgson Mill®. I usually sprinkle a tablespoon of it on my oatmeal or Cream of Wheat®.

"Life is not complex. We are complex. Life is simple, and the simple thing is the right thing."–Oscar Wilde

ProGreens by Nutricology®

ProGreens by Nutricology® is a synthesis of some of the best nutrients that nature has ever provided in an amazing green powder. This green powder is mixed with juice or with water and drunk in the morning on an empty stomach for best absorption, though you can take it at any time of the day. This powder mixed and drunk on a regular basis affords for you so many benefits that I will have to take the next fours pages just to show you what it contains and what each nutrient does for you. For one thing amongst others, you can say goodbye to stomach bloat and constipation, probably within the first couple of weeks. You will sleep better. Your energy will go up. You will feel in better moods. You will feel less the effects of stress. Your body will metabolize better. And you might even notice an improvement in your sex life.

After I have had my vigorous morning workout, I will go in and mix a scoop of this magic green powder with water and orange Crystal Light® just before I have breafast. The minute I do, it is as though I feel the positive action on my body working instantly. Maybe it's just my imagination. Who knows. Who cares! It's a consistent feeling, so I have no reason to give up on this daily health routine.

In the next four pages, I will break down in even greater detail all of the nutrients and what they do that is listed on the jars of ProGreens.

ProGreens®

Nutrient	Amount	%Daily	Action
Protein	2 g	4%	Builds muscle tissue
Vitamin A	670 IU	13%	Eye health and function
Vitamin C	16 mg	27%	Skin Health
Vitamin E	100 IU	330%	• Contributes to heart health, mental and prostate health.
Calcium	29 mg	3%	Healthy bones
Iron	1.8 mg	10%	• Carry life-giving oxygen to human blood cells.
Wheat grass powder	350 mg	†	• Cleanses the blood and increases red blood cell count. Stimulates metabolism.
Barley grass powder	350 mg	†	• Barley Grass contains a most amazing nutrients "Chlorophyll "(Liquid Oxygenated Sunshine), a detoxifier that rids the intestines of stored toxins.
Alfalfa grass powder	350 mg	†	• Plays as an effective controller of cholesterol.
Oat grass powder	350 mg	†	• Contains beta-carotene, vitamins K and C, folic acid, calcium, iron, protein, fiber and B vitamins.
Spirulina	1,000 mg	†	• Spirulina provides all the required amino acids, and in a form that is five times easier to digest than meat or soy protein.
Chlorella (cracked cell)	350 mg	†	• Improves the digestive system and decreases constipation. Chlorella speeds up bowel, bloodstream and liver cleansing by supplying chlorophyll.

Nutrient	Amount	%Daily	Action	ProGreens®
Dunaliella salina	40 mg	†	• Reinforces the immune system, and slows down aging and cell degradation. May help to prevent cerebral tumors, leukemia, skin, liver and stomach cancers.	
Nova Scotia Dulse	30 mg	†	• Dulse may help reverse hardening of the arteries, reduce high blood pressure, regress and prevent tumors.	
Licorice root powder	100 mg	†	• Flavonoids of the licorice plant have been shown to kill Helicobacter pylori, the bacteria causing most ulcers and stomach inflammation.	
Siberian Ginseng	60 mg	†	• Invigorates the entire body and aides the immune system.	
Pfaffia Paniculata	60 mg	†	• May restore sexual function in both men and women.	
Astragalus	60 mg	†	• A potent tonic for increasing energy levels and stimulating the immune system.	
Echinacea purpurea	60 mg	†	• Stimulates the white blood cells, fighting colds and flu as well as boosts the lymphatic system.	
Ginger root powder	5 mg	†	• Can be used for treating such ailments as common colds, flu, headache, motion sickness and athlete's foot.	

Nutrient	Amount	%Daily	Action	**ProGreens®**
Soy Lecithin (99% oil-free)	2,000 mg	†	• Believed to be beneficial for treating high cholesterol, anxiety, and liver disease.	
Acerola berry juice powder	200 mg	†	• Acerola Berry Juice powder provides a rich natural source of Vitamin C .	
Beet juice powder	200 mg	†	• Betaine, an amino acid in beet root, has significant anti-cancer properties. Studies show that beet juice inhibits formation of cancer-causing compounds in the colon.	
Spinach octacosanol	150 mg	†	• A nutrient promoting stamina and energy.	
Royal jelly (5% 10-HDA)	150 mg	†	• Can help to lower cholesterol.	
Bee pollen	150 mg	†	• Bee pollen helps build resistance to allergies.	
Flaxseed meal	500 mg	†	• Aides the digestion, regulates the bowels and aides in metabolizing fat cells.	
Apple pectin & fiber	500 mg	†	• Apple pectin is helpful in maintaining good digestive health.	

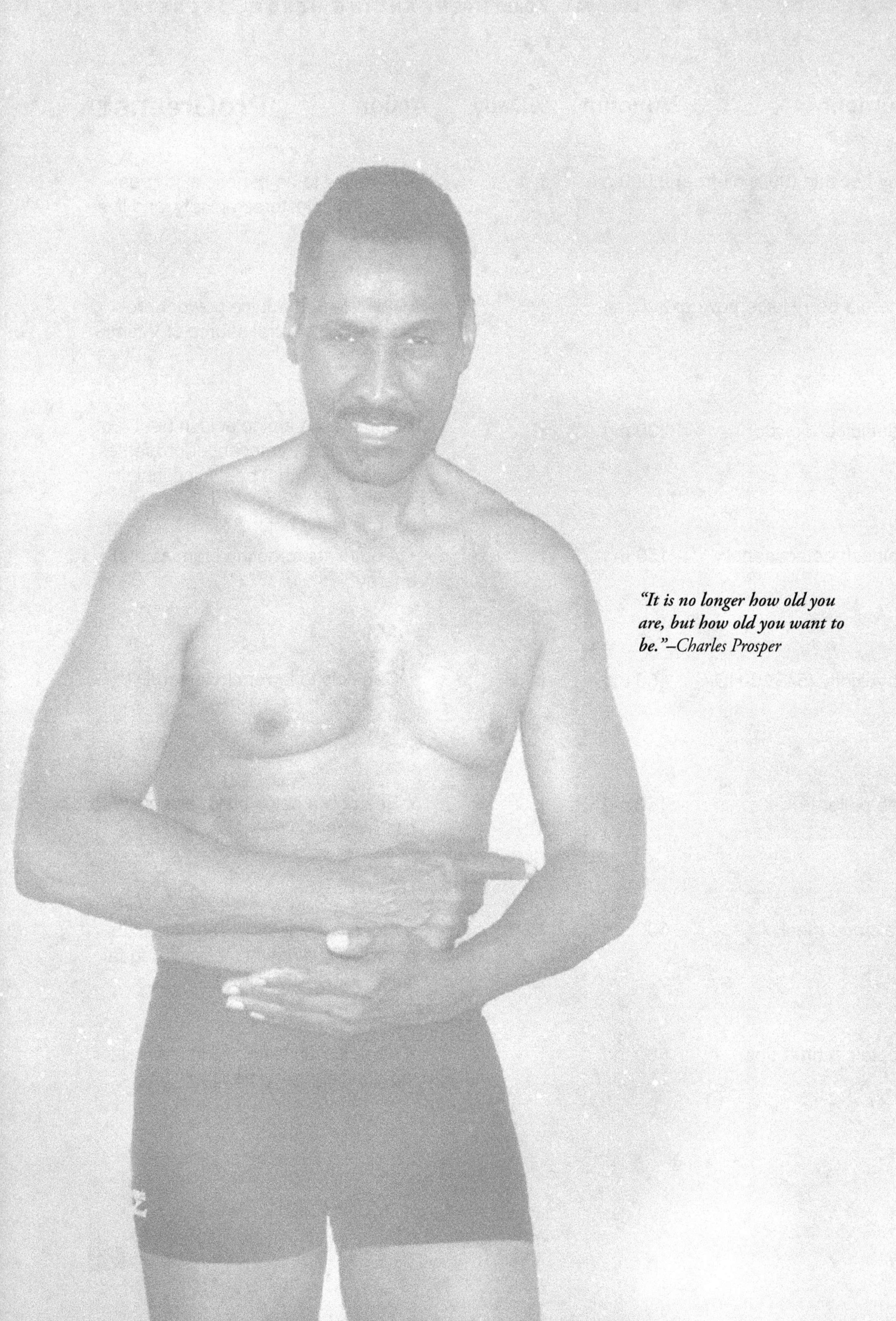

"It is no longer how old you are, but how old you want to be."–Charles Prosper

CHAPTER 13

An Interview with Bernie Long – 68-Year Young Fountain of Youth

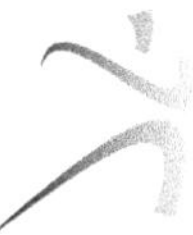

"Strength is a matter of the made-up mind."–John Beecher

As they say, a picture is worth a thousands words, and this impressive photo of 68-year young hunk says it all. Is there any doubt as to what is possible if you have the correct method and put your mind to it?

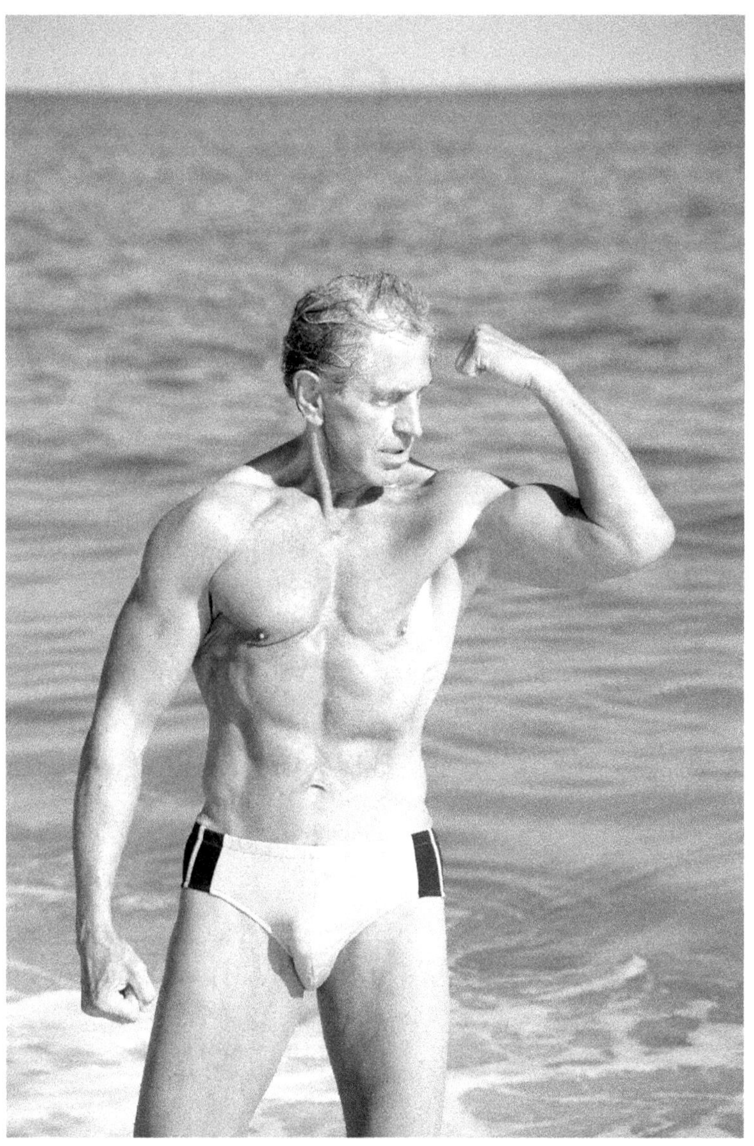

Mr. Bernie Long (68 years young)

Photography by Rob Lang

Q: Well, I am very excited to be on the phone live talking with Mr. Bernie Long, the Fountain of Youth, or as I saw him in Exercise For Men Only *as Mr. Longevity.* I was totally blown away when I saw this young man of 68 years old. I couldn't believe my eyes. How're you doing today, Bernie?

B.L. I'm terrific, thank you.

Q: You know, when I first saw you in the November 2009 issue of Exercise For Men Only, I was totally blown away by how you look. You look like a man of 30, 20.... I know some kids in their twenties that don't look as good as you do.

B.L. *(Laugther.)*

Q: And when I saw your story, I said: "My God! Bernie follows some of the same principles that I advocate and espouse in my book!" And I said to myself: "I've *got* to get an interview with Bernie! I don't know what it's going to take, but I've got to get an interview with this man." So, here we are. Bernie, there are a lot of people that are very excited to hear about your story. The thing I want to ask you is just this point. What got you so dedicated to physical fitness and to look so good, so darn good at 68?

"It's an ill plan that cannot be changed."–Latin proverb

B.L. Well, actually, I had always worked out, and have done lots of different things. At one point I was doing a lot of swimming. I had a swimming coach. And at another point, I was doing a lot of cycling, and I had a cycling coach. But I think what brought me to the point where I really wanted to put a lot of effort into exercising and really focus on it happened when I was about 59 years of age. I had a series of mini-strokes that....

Q: You mean heart attacks?

B.L. No, no, these were in the brain.

Q: Oh!

B.L. They were mini-strokes that left me with some memory loss, an inability to do multifunctional tasks and that kind of thing....

Q: Um hum!

B.L. And I had to stop working and go on permanent disability. This was a very disruptive and disturbing time in my life.

Q: Now were you in good physical shape at this time?

B.L. Yes, I was in reasonably good shape. These mini-strokes were not the result of poor health condition. Initially, my doctors thought they were caused by an opening between the two upper chambers of the heart that didn't close at birth. Finally they decided that these strokes most likely were caused by a cerebral vasculitis.

Q: And so, how did this relate to your change as for your physical goals and your health goal?

B.L. Well, first of all, I had certainly lots of time on my hands, and once I had recovered to some degree from the disorder and disruption in my life (depression and that kind of thing), I began to try to reclaim my sense of self and re-establish myself. One of the things I did was I started working out with Scott Weisse at the gym.

Q: And I know you have praised Scott Weisse highly as being pivotal in helping you get into the amazing shape that you are in today. Isn't that right?

"The death of dogma is the birth of reality."–Immanuel Kant

B.L. Yes, indeed he has. He's amazing because it's like he doesn't start out with, "We have this colossal program we need to achieve." It's more like, "Let's work on this effort and we'll build on it as you improve."

Q: Um Hum.

B.L. Like, one of the things I can remember now, which probably was about five years ago, he said, "Okay, we're going to have you learn how to do 100 push ups." I thought, "Jesus, 100 push ups. I can't do 10."

Q: Um Hum.

B.L. Well, I learned how to do 100 push ups! And he made it into a little competitive thing. With each session, I would do a little bit more. And he would vary the routine. Not just the same old thing. We might vary the number of sets or number of reps per set.

Q: And how old were you at that point?

B.L. I had to be about 63.

Q: Wow!

B.L. Mostly all of this working out with Scott and with weights started at 63 onwards.

Q: Really!

B.L. Yes.

Q: If you want to hear something funny, Bernie, my barber, the guy who cuts my hair – he said to me, and he's a little out of shape, so he's getting into cycling, "I need to do something because I'm getting a little old." And you know how old he is? Mid-thirties.

B.L. *(Laughter.)*

Q: I said: "Look, you're talking to the wrong person if you want sympathy from me. *(Laughter.)* Mid-thirties, come on!

"Do the thing you fear, and the death of fear is certain."– Ralph Waldo Emerson

B.L. I think it's very smart that your barber thinks this way. Scott has said things like that to me. Scott is 45, but he already realizes what the aging process can do if you don't do something to resist and counteract it.

Q: Would you agree...? I have this saying that "Before 30, youth is God's gift to you. And after 30, youth is your gift to yourself."

B.L. Indeed it is. I think that I didn't realize this as wholeheartedly as I do now...until after I'd had my mini-strokes. And it's amazing. I think sometimes it does take a real jolt in our lives to bring into focus those things that are truly important...to us. And I think that's what really happened to me. It made me realize there's no reason why I can't do many of the things that, physically, I felt I couldn't do before. And Scott certainly has been a great coach in helping me challenge these preconceived notions.

Q: Now your advice. My particular passion or niche is focusing on the baby boomers, the people who have past 40 and are reaching 50, and thinking it's over and it's too late. What is you advice to the person in terms of is it ever too late to start?

B.L. It's *never* too late to start. Never! And, I think that it is important not to start out by establishing big colossal goals to achieve. You're simply going to go to the gym. And if you can't even get on a bike and warm up properly, you're going to learn how to do that. That may be the first thing that you learn. And then you build from there. Scott has taught me how to challenge myself and train to do more reps of any given exercise. As I mentioned, early on I learned how to do 100 push-ups. And then from there we went to curls. And from there we went to dips. And from there we went to pull-ups and chin-ups. ...and I'm not talking about doing five or ten, but multiple sets of 10s and 15s.

Q: Now, you're 68. How many push-ups can you do now?

B.L. Right now, I could *easily* do a set of 25, then rest and do another 25.

Q: Wow!

B.L. To do 100 push-ups, I would have to work up to that again. But I could do it. I'd have to re-train the body. If you don't do it, you lose it. And the older you get, the quicker you lose it.

"Success comes before work only in the dictionary."– Anonymous

Q: That's amazing!

B.L. When I started out, I couldn't do one pull-up, one-chin up. Now, I could *easily* do 10 at a time.

Q: If you woke up tomorrow and didn't know your age, let's say you had some kind of age amnesia, and you didn't actually even look at yourself in the mirror, how old would you say you are based on how you feel?

B.L. Humm. I'm not going to answer that just the way you asked it. *(Laughter.)* Instead, let's say I'm going to be able to look in the mirror. So, if I'm able to look in the mirror...I'd say I could be...45, or maybe 40.

Q: I would agree with that – wholeheartedly.

B.L. I mean, I feel that way when I look into the mirror. I don't feel *"old"!* I don't feel 68. And, actually, I'll be 69 in a few months.

Q: Wow! That's amazing! Now, the subtitle of my book "How To Get Fit Fast At Any Age" is "It is no longer how old you are but

how old you want to be." And a lot a people don't realize that they have a lot of say-so in how old they want to be. Chronologically, we can't stop the movement of time, but physiologically, I do believe, and you're proof of that for me, that we can reverse the aging process and return to the point where we're *physiologically 40 at 70 years old.* Would you agree?

B.L. I definitely agree. And indeed you can.

Q: Now, I've noticed this, and a lot of people have asked me this. When I put up your picture on Facebook, and I started talking about the book, and there was one person that asked me, and I pretty much know your answer even before I ask you, but I want to have *you* give it to me. He asked me: "Is diet involved? Are eating habits involved?" And so, the question is, what is your eating philosophy? Do you believe in the big, three square meals a day?

B.L. No. Not at all.

Q: Okay, tell us?

"If you start to take Vienna, take Vienna."–Napoleon Bonaparte

B.L. Again, something I've learned from Scott is, it's better to have small meals. I have 6 small meals a day.

Q: With what frequency? How many hours in between each meal?

B.L. Well, you all have to get them in during your waking hours, and you should try to get 8 hours of sleep, if at all possible. That means you have 16 hours to work with. One thing that I do which doesn't allow me to cheat is that I record everything that I eat over the course of each day on my computer. I put in the proteins, carbohydrates, fats, calories – and total it up. I'm not a slave to the totals or anything like that, but it's a wonderful mechanism for going back and reviewing what I've eaten over any period of time. For example, if I put on 3 or 4 lbs., I didn't put on 3 or 4 lbs. by accident – something happened. I probably changed my diet in some way. This way, I can go back and revise what I am doing. Like today, I'm 192 lbs. with a 33-inch waist – which is basically my ideal bodyweight.

Q: Now let me ask you this, for the sake of people that really want to know, and who are detailed-oriented like myself. Give us briefly a run of typical day of what you would eat. Give us a run of a typical day, for example, if you get up at, say, 7:00 a.m. or at 9:00 a.m. what would you eat?

B.L. As soon as I get up in the morning, the first thing I do is, I take my medications. Next, I weigh myself, and I measure my waist. I record my weight and waist measurement in my Palm Pilot. I have been doing that for the last five or six years. And then the next thing I do are some stretches. I have certain stretches that I do every morning before I do anything, and it's the last thing I do before I go to bed at night. After showering and shaving, I go out to Starbucks every morning where I have a large cup of black coffee and a cinnamon chip scone...

Q: Now, wait a minute, Bernie. I'm a southern boy from New Orleans. We don't eat scones down there? What the heck is a scone?

B.L. *(Laughter.)* A scone is like a small biscuit that is made with cream and eggs and is cut into diamond shapes and baked in an oven or on a griddle.

Q: Oh, okay.

"The secret to success in any human endeavor is total concentration."–Kurt Vonnegut

B.L. *(Laughter.)* And that's my first meal of the day. And it's probably somewhat luxurious because it's not considered a weight or calorie-conscious type of thing.

Q: Now, is this about an hour or two later?

B.L. Yes, that's about right.

Q: So, that first meal was about what time? Give us a rough idea.

B.L. Oh, it could be nine o'clock in the morning.

Q: Okay, and then the next meal is about twelve.

B.L. About twelve.

Q: Okay, now tell us what you eat at that meal. Go ahead.

B.L. Then I have two hard-boiled eggs. That's it.

Q: With the yolk?

B.L. With the yolk - indeed I do.

Q: Okay.

B.L. And then from there...

Q: Was that it?

B.L. Yes, that's it, for that meal.

Q: Any water? Any drink?

B.L. Oh, yes, I have a glass of water when I take my daily vitamins and supplements at this time.

"To do two things at once is to do neither."–*Publilius Syrus*

Q: Alright, now we're at noon...

B.L. We're at noon, and I usually, let's say on workout days, I'm going off to the gym. I will have an energy drink during my workout and a muscle-building drink immediately following my workout.

Q: Now, what time is this, Bernie?

B.L. That could be anywhere from 3:00 to 5:00 in the afternoon. Like today, it'll be 4:00 o'clock.

Q: Now, you drink this before or during your workout?

B.L. I have something that I take during the workout, and then I also have a post-workout drink.

Q: Now, tell us what that drink is.

B.L. The energy drink that I take during the workout is called Super Pump 250. And then I also have a post-workout drink called Surge, which is a muscle-building energy drink.

Q: I see, these are your drinks pre and post workout.

B.L. Actually, it's *during* and *after* my workout.

Q: Now, this doesn't give your stomach queasiness?

B.L. No, absolutely not.

Q: Okay.

B.L. No, if it did, I wouldn't use it.

Q: Of course, that's obvious.

B.L. At times, Scott varies the drinks that I have. So, at a different time, it may be a different kind of drink. But I am always having something during and after. And then, usually, about 6:00 o'clock in the evening, I will stop off at this wonderful takeout place across the street from me. And I'll get a grilled salmon.

"Each man is capable of doing one thing well. If he attempts several, he will fail to achieve distinction in any."–Plato

Q: And what else?

B.L. That's it. Just a grilled salmon.

Q: No vegetables?

B.L. No, not at this time.

Q: Do you eat vegetables at all?

B.L. Oh, yes. Yes, indeed. So then, comes dinner time.

Q: And what time is that?

B.L. What I call dinner is usually 8:00 or 9:00 o'clock at night, I will have two *big* iced teas, unsweetened because I don't like sugar in iced tea. Also, I will have a green salad, and two breasts of chicken with a double order of steamed broccoli, because adding mashed potatoes can cause me to gain weight.

I have learned to *love* steamed broccoli. So, I'll have that, and that's my dinner, and it's a huge meal. And then, just before I go to bed....

Q: What time is that?

B.L. That would be about 11:30 at night before I go to bed, I will have a low-carb protein shake called Metabolic Drive.

Q: Now, let me ask you this, Bernie. I believe in this kind of eating. I eat five times a day; you eat six. Now, this is what I want to ask you. I have a "cheat day". Like on Sundays, I eat whatever I want. Do you have a "cheat day"?

B.L. I don't have a "cheat day," but I definitely have "cheat meals." And, not on any particular day. I can't be slavish to anything. And when I cheat, I really cheat. There's a restaurant that I love to go to, over on the Westside. It's called "Good Enough To Eat".

Q: *(Laughter.)*

"The first law of success...is concentration: to bend all the energies to one point, and to to directly to that point, looking neither to the right nor the left."–William Matthews

B.L. And I go there usually once a week. It's often on a Saturday night. I always start off with two iced teas, a green salad and lightly-grilled cornbread. Then my main course might be meat loaf with ketchup, mashed potatoes, peas and carrots. And then I'll always top off dinner with (which is one of the reasons I go to this restaurant) with one of their incredible desserts.

Q: Now, what dessert does Bernie Long eat? Tell us.

B.L. Well, I'll have a giant piece of coconut cake. Last time I was there, I had a big piece of German chocolate cake.

Q: Oh, my goodness. Okay.

B.L. But they have all kinds of wonderful, very gloppy desserts. And I have *no* idea how many calories...or what's in it. I just note it in my diary, and don't try to calculate how many calories. *(Laugther.)*

Q: Well, you know what I have found? I have found this, Bernie. It's that you body adjusts to that irregularity. In fact, I have noticed that on my "cheat day", I actually feel my body heating up as though my metabolism was saying, "Whoops, something is wrong here. This is not supposed to be coming in. Let's speed things up." So, I believe that your metabolism actually speeds up on your "cheat day" to accomodate for that difference which is irregular to what your

body is used to.

B.L. Interesting. I never even thought of that, but I think of it more from an emotional point of view. I think that with any of these things, you can't be too restrictive and too rigid about it. For one thing, with my way of life, I eat out with friends all of the time. You know, it just wouldn't work. They would be bored to tears if they had to go to always to the same kinds of restaurants with me just to satisfy my needs.

Q: Exactly. Exactly. Now, we want to definitely get this question in. What is your exercise philosophy? Is it aerobics only à-la-Richard Simmons? Is it progressive weight resistance? Is it pilates? How do *you* exercise? Do you lift weights? Do you do aerobics? What's your philosophy?

B.L. The primary focus of my workouts is on strengthening and conditioning my entire body, in addition to improving my energy system fitness. Whenever possible, Scott believes an exercise should be functional, that is, mimicking tasks/movements of everyday life. Following through on this workout theory, we seldom use exercise machines. Instead, we use free weights, pulley weight, gymnastic rings, pull-up bars, rubber bands, kettle bells, sand bags, abdominal wheel and weighted Prowler sled.

"A single idea, if it is right, saves us the labor of an infinity of experiences."–Jacques Maritain

Q: Good. Okay.

B.L. My workouts frequently incorporate bodyweight training, using added weights or added resistance. The exercises vary from simple movements to compound body movements. Scott includes exercises specifically geared to improve flexibility, coordination or stability which, at the same time, build muscular strength.

Q: So, the answer is yes, that you do use weights and progressive resistance. Do you do a separate type of exercises just for aerobics? Or are your weight resistance exercises incorporating aerobic activity?

B.L. They include an aerobic element. What I mean is that if you're going through a circuit or multiple sets, for example, it's all timed, and that's incredible because it really pushes you. As soon as the time is up, you've got to move to the next exercise or next set. You get a short rest, but it's not one where you're energy systems come down to a resting state. Not at all, you keep right on going. Yes, it's highly aerobic.

Q: Now, is weight training also good for women?

B.L. I think it's very good. One of the things you showed me, which I thought was just extraordinary was that woman.... How old was she? 71 or so?

Q: 87.

B.L. 87!! *(Exclaiming)* I looked at her on YouTube. I think it's sensational. I looked at her, and it didn't matter so much about her physicality.... What I was so impressed by was her stature. I mean the woman stands so damned erect that you would think she was 21 years of age. It's wonderful to see.

Q: And she started when she was 73. She is one of my heroes as well, Marjorie Newlin. I have a mantel piece of heroes. On it is Marjorie Newlin, Bernie Long, you know and a select few....

B.L. Well, I think she is wonderful. All I can say, again, is that anyone at that age who can stand up and move like she is in her twenties or thirties is just sensational.

"Great works are performed not by strength, but by perseverance."–Samuel Johnson

Q: So, Bernie, we're wrapping things up right now. This has really been exciting and interesting just to go into your world and your mind. Any last words of advice or encouragement for those people out there who are in their fifties or sixties, and they are wondering if it is all over? What are your last words of advice for us?

B.L. Well, first of all, it's not all over. Not at all - in no way. And I think the thing that one has to keep in mind is this...and again I go back to something I said earlier, which is...you know, it can be very intimidating and very threatening for someone who hasn't been in the gym for many years or maybe never - to even think about going to the gym. My advice is don't think about how colossal all of this is going to be. Just get there. And take it one step at a time.

Q: It doesn't matter how weak you are to begin?

B.L. No. Not at *all!* Because if you have a good trainer, that trainer is going to find something that you can do that is going to be a challenge for you *as you are today*. Then you start on that, and you build on it. And if you really are committed to it, you will make progress, and as you make progress, that will excite you more. And make you want to do even more.

Q: As we are wrapping up, I know that you want to get some information to the people who might want to get in contact with you, because you are amongst other things a fitness model, so what is your website?

B.L. My website is `www.BernieLong.com`.

Q: And you are in the New York City area?

B.L. Yes, that is correct. I live in Manhattan. On my website, I have a contact form where you can contact me by email.

Q: And I know you have spoken highly of Scott Weisse. If someone is in the New York area and they want to get in contact with a good fitness trainer, how would they get in contact with Scott.

"Victory belongs to the most perservering."–Napoleon Bonaparte

B.L. His E-mail is `ScottWeisse@yahoo.com`

Q: Well, Mr. Bernie Long, it's been a pleasure, an honor and a privilege. You are one of my heroes. I want to be like you when I grow up.

B.L. *(Laughter. Much laughter.)* Thank you so much.

Q: *(Continued laughter.)* It's been a pleasure talking to you, and until the next time.

B.L. And likewise, until the next time.

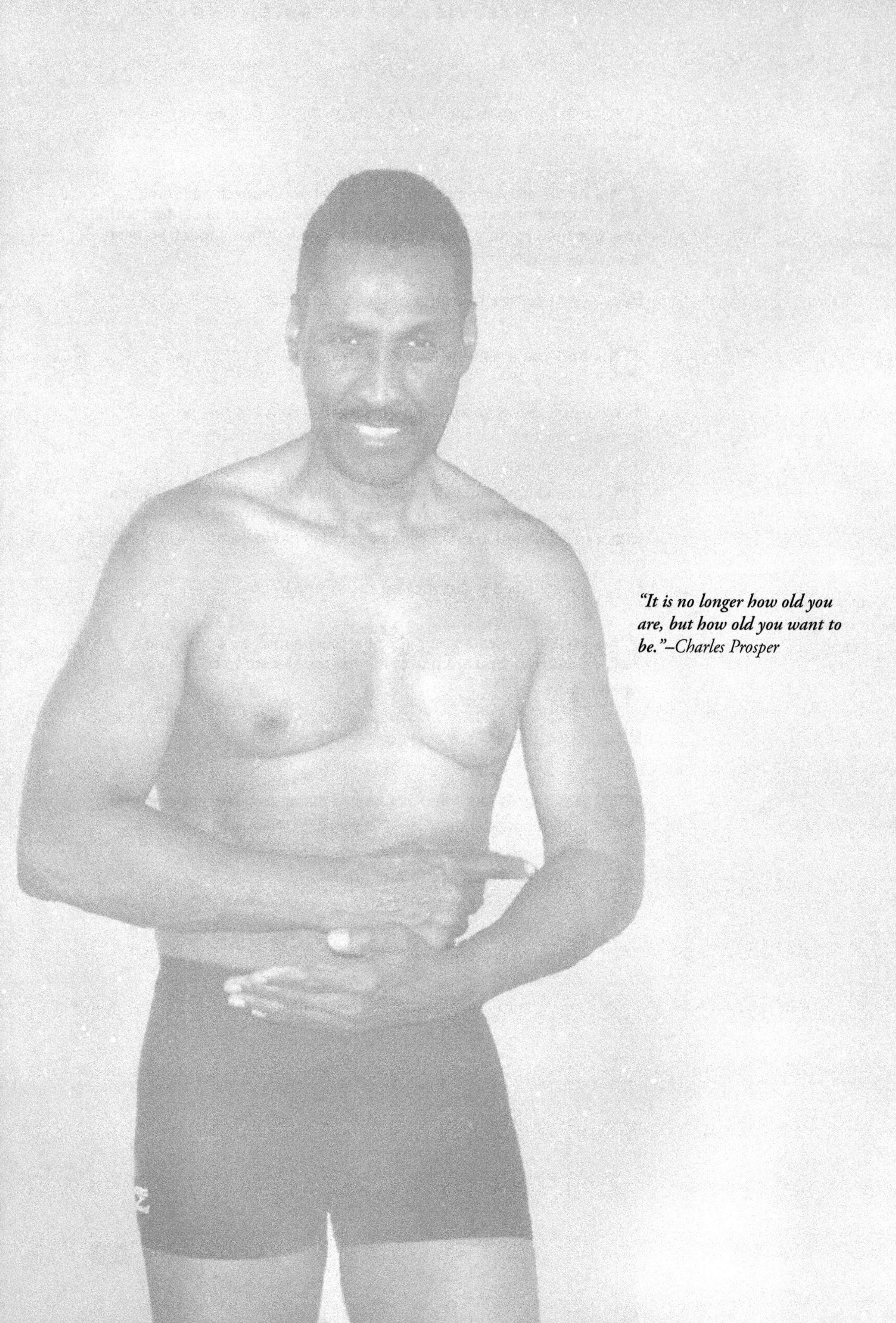

"It is no longer how old you are, but how old you want to be."–Charles Prosper

Why This Book Is For Women In Their 40's

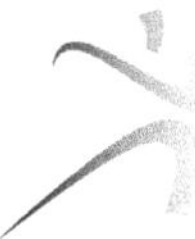

Denise Brideau Kenny is a black belt in karate and a star athlete who, at 47, has the strength, fitness, flexibility and agility of a woman in her 20's. In this interview, Denise teaches women here how to be young.

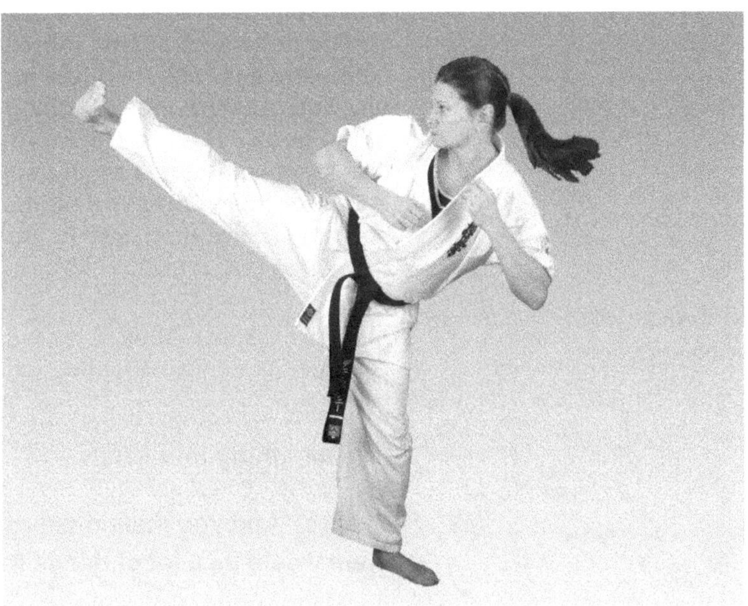

Denise Kenny (Fit at 47)

Photography by Donald Rail - Hourglass Fotografi

Charles: **Well, this is yours truly, Charles Prosper, and I am interviewing my good friend, colleague, and proofreader, Denise Kenny. How are you doing tonight, Denise?**

Den: I'm great, Charles. And you?

Charles: **Okay. Fine. I just want to introduce the readers to you in the fact that, I know you are a little shy about this, but nevertheless, I think you are quite an accomplished athlete, and you can speak with authority on what we're going to talk about tonight. You have a black belt in something. What is it? Can you tell us?**

Den: Kyokushin Kai (Karate).

Charles: **And you have been doing this for how long now?**

Den: 8 years exactly.

Charles: **8 years, okay. And I've seen some of the kicks that you have had, and the pictures, and you look like you're made out of nothing but elastic. *(Laughter.)* The first time I saw you with a kick so high I said: "Okay, where's the string that's holding up your leg?" *(Laughter.)***

Den: *(Laughter.)* No strings attached.

Charles: **Now, you have been in a very unusual position of being not only my proofreader for my book, which I really, really appreciate. You've done a smashing job, but also the fact that you're my friend colleague and fellow-athlete in your own right whom I admire quite a bit. You pointed out something to me. As you were reading the title of the book, "How To Get Fit At Any Age", you made mention to me that it may confuse a lot of people, for example women, that this book is not for them. And you pointed out that that's not the case. Would you say that women, and in particular women in their 30's and just barely making it to their 40's, could benefit from the book as well?**

"Do whatever you do intensely."–Robert Henri

Den: Of course. Well, I started training basically in karate 8 years ago. I was 40 years old. And I just needed to get in shape. And this book would have been perfect at the time, had it been published. I just happened to jump into karate.

Charles: **And you mentioned to me after you read it, you saw how there would be a lot of things in there that you could use even now.**

Den: Yes, because we have the same need as men do, and we also want a nice body. So, why not?

Charles: **And the thing is that I kind of focused on this niche when I put the over fifty thing, and I did this with a lot of consideration because most of the people, once you hit the mid-century mark, you get a lot of people that give up, and they start whining and complaining. And the thing is this. I believe women in particular need to understand how important it is because women are very prone to osteoporosis. The bones get brittle after age 40.**

Den: And it's proven that when you keep fit, these problems hardly appear for your age group of 60, 70 or higher because you take care of yourself. You eat well. You exercise. It's a life style. And women need that as much as men do. And when I saw the Fifty, I thought, gees, I'm not there yet, but at forty, I already needed that, and I know that women under forty have the same needs. Most women take care of the household, the kids, and then yourself. You don't exercise because you don't see the time. You can't seem to find the time until you start.

Charles: **Until you start deteriorating, you have all that time for the doctor visits. *(Laughter.)* And this starts to hurt, and that starts to hurt...Den, do you remember that article that I sent you of that lady, Marjorie Newlin, who lifts weights and takes care of herself so superbly at 87 years old?**

Den: Yep, I do. I'm going to be just like her at that age. *(Laughter.)*

Charles: ***(Continued laughter.)* Yeah, why not? And you know how old she was when she started?**

Den: How old?

Charles: **Or how young she was, I should say...She was 73 years old.**

Den: You see, that's the problem. Most people think you can't start at 40, 50, even older. You think you have to be 20 to be in shape. That's a misconception. Totally. I'm in better shape today, and I'm going on 48, than I was at 30.

"One thought driven home is better than three left on base."–James Liter

Charles: **Wow!**

Den: Because I wanted to. It's never too late.

Charles: **And that's the message. I'm so glad you said that. That is definitely the message. It's never too late. Because the thing is, I have met many people who are in their 50's and they look like they're in their 70's. You know, something happens. It's like there is a mental shift in people when they hit a certain age. You want to hear something funny? I told Bernie Long this, the other gentleman who's in the book, who's going to be 69 and this guy looks like 39...Did you see his picture?**

Den: He's incredible!

Charles: **Yeah, he is! He is 68 and has the body of a gymnast of 30. He could do 100 pushups.**

Den: A lot of young people can't do that!

Charles: **Of course not. And the thing is, I have noticed that you become old when you decide to become old.**

Den: It's all in your head.

Charles: **Exactly. My barber who is, I think, 33, told me the other day when he was cutting my hair: "You know, Charles, I'm getting old."** ***(Laughter.)*** **I said: "Excuse me!"** ***(More laughter.)*** **I said: "You're talking to the wrong person if you want sympathy."** ***(More laughter.)*** **And also I remember that I made a decision when I was 25. My decision was, I'm not going to ever let an old man move into this body. That was my decision, and I've kept my word...And I will never, ever, ever, and I would suggest to anyone to do the same, male or female, to ever say to yourself, "I'm getting old." You will never hear me say that! I would never say that even in joking because you are setting yourself up to go that route even faster.**

Den: And you follow it. I think these people need motivation and that is what's missing a lot. You look at Bernie Long, and you say: "Oh my gosh, how could I get that body!" Anybody can do that.

Charles: **Or you look at Marjorie Newlin, the 87 year old lady.**

Den: Same thing, same thing. Anybody can do it. A lot of people ask me at karate, parents, mothers, "How do you do it?" And I tell them, I started just to be with my girls, to do the sport. "You can do it too!" I wasn't born this way. I had to work at it. Things weren't always the way they are now. I was overweight for a while. I had about 30 pounds too much on me.

"Only a weak mind seeks ultimate answers."–Agnes Thornton

Charles: **When was this?**

Den: My eldest was born in 1991, and the other in 1994. So, that was about in 1996 or 1997. So, almost thirteen years ago. I was about 30 pounds overweight. And I felt like I was too old. And I was already in shape before. I used to run when I was in school. I was on the track team and stuff like that.

Charles: **Um Hum.**

Den: But I never, never in my wildest dreams thought I would go and do karate or anything like that. I was a mommy. That's it. And a working mommy at that. But when they started karate, I was there all the time, so the Sensei told me. She said: "You should start the classes with them. You look good, and you could do well." And gees, I went to Canadian championships, U.S. Open, and I won everything because I was capable, and I got into shape...You need a passion! Once you've got that*(Pause)*...I wasn't fifty any more...I was twenty! *(Laughter.)*

Charles: **Um Hum.**

Den: Things happen when you want things to happen. And I love the cover of the book. I love the color. And I just had a few comments that I wrote down that I had to tell you.

Charles: **Good.**

Den: Yes, after forty, when you're a woman, you don't feel as good about yourself as you used to. That's normal. But when you start doing something...I started karate at forty. It just happened that way. Today I'm almost fifty, and I'm like 25 or 30. I go to class, and I'm the oldest one there. All the kids, they all look up to me...young adults, young guys, young girls. And I'm like the mommy there, but I'm mostly like a big sister to them.

Charles: **So that's the thing, you decided to become young, and you became young.**

Den: Yep, and you're not that old person anymore. My mom at 40... to me, she was like 60, physically. She was not a physically fit person at 40. She was home all day. She wasn't working. She was doing home stuff. In those days, mothers were not active like we are today.

"In doubt, fear is the worst of prophets."–Statius

Charles: **And they aged much faster.**

Den: Well, yes. Well look at Bernie Long, my God, I can hardly believe it. He's 68 and has a great body!

Charles: **The thing is that there have been very few role models that we could see it was possible. The reason why we give up, at, say 40, is because we've never seen a Bernie Long. We've never seen a Marjorie Newlin who started bodybuilding, lifting weights at 73 and went on to win fitness contests at 87 donning a two-piece bikini! We don't even think that they can exist. With this book, I hope to expand people's consciousness to the fact that there is that potential.**

Den: And the thing is also, like in sports, hockey players, they retire at 40. Athletes are too old after 25, 26 to go to the Olympics, depending on which sport. But most athletes retire at 40, like baseball players, if they're over 40, they're a legend.

Charles: **And that starts that programming in a person's mind.**

Den: Like in karate, the last two or three years, I used to compete with the younger people. And now I'm with the over-40 category. I used to be the only person over 40 who would compete because I was the only woman who was in shape enough over here. Like, I had to compete against women in their twenties, and I had the cardio...

Charles: **Chronologically, you can't stop the years, but physiologically, you are a young mama. *(Laughter.)***

Den: Yes, yes, because everywhere I go in competition, they don't think that I'm that old. They think I'm in my late thirties. That's a plus for me.

Charles: **Den, the message here, and the reason why I had you here is just to talk to you about this, and drive home that this book is for women. It is definitely for women. And it's for women in their 20's, in their 30's, in their 40's – at any stage that you wish. I had to chose some title, and I picked on a certain group, but I really want to open the doors to all. In fact, tomorrow, I have my neighbor who works out with me in my garden; he's going to give me an interview because I have shown him some of my techniques, and he's 31. He's found that everything that I've shown him works for him as well. So, the information in here is not age-specific. It's a catchy title that gets the attention of those who think it is over.**

"If you think too long, you think wrong."–Jim Kaat

Den: When I read your book and saw your program, I was just amazed. It's really good. You don't have to be a man. You don't have to be fifty.

Charles: **And it works extremely well for women, as soon as they realize it's the right time to start. The moment you realize it, is the right time to start. And you, Den, I've seen the condition that you're in, and you're absolutely in superb condition. I was shocked just now when you told me 47. I was thinking 37.**

Den: I'll be 48 in July.

Charles: **You see that's the thing about people, men and women, who take care of themselves, they remove physiologically decades off their bodies.**

Den: Yep, indeed.

Charles: **And that's what we have to realize. It's never too late. And the whole mantra, and theme of my book is: "It is no longer how old you are, but how old you want to be." And everybody has to ask, "How old do I really want to be?" And you're not going to get sympathy from Marjorie Newlin. *(Laughter.)* You're not going to get sympathy from Bernie Long.**

Den: No, and not from me either, and not from you.

Charles: ***(Laughter.)*** **And not from me. Not when the path to health and fitness has been laid out quite nicely. So, basically, this just has been our little chit-chat, so we can get that message out, and have people understand. So, if you happen to be flipping through the book right now, know, that at whatever stage you are, 20, 30, 40, 50, 60 or 70, or above, that the things that we have here in this book are definitely for you. And so, I just want to thank you my good friend, and because you're in karate, let me see, how shall I end this...just keep on kickin'.**

Den: Alright. OSU! *(Laughter.)*

Charles: ***(Continued laughter.)*** **Okay, we thank you so much, and until the next time.**

Den: You're very welcome.

"We cannot solve life's problems except by solving them."–M. Scott Peck

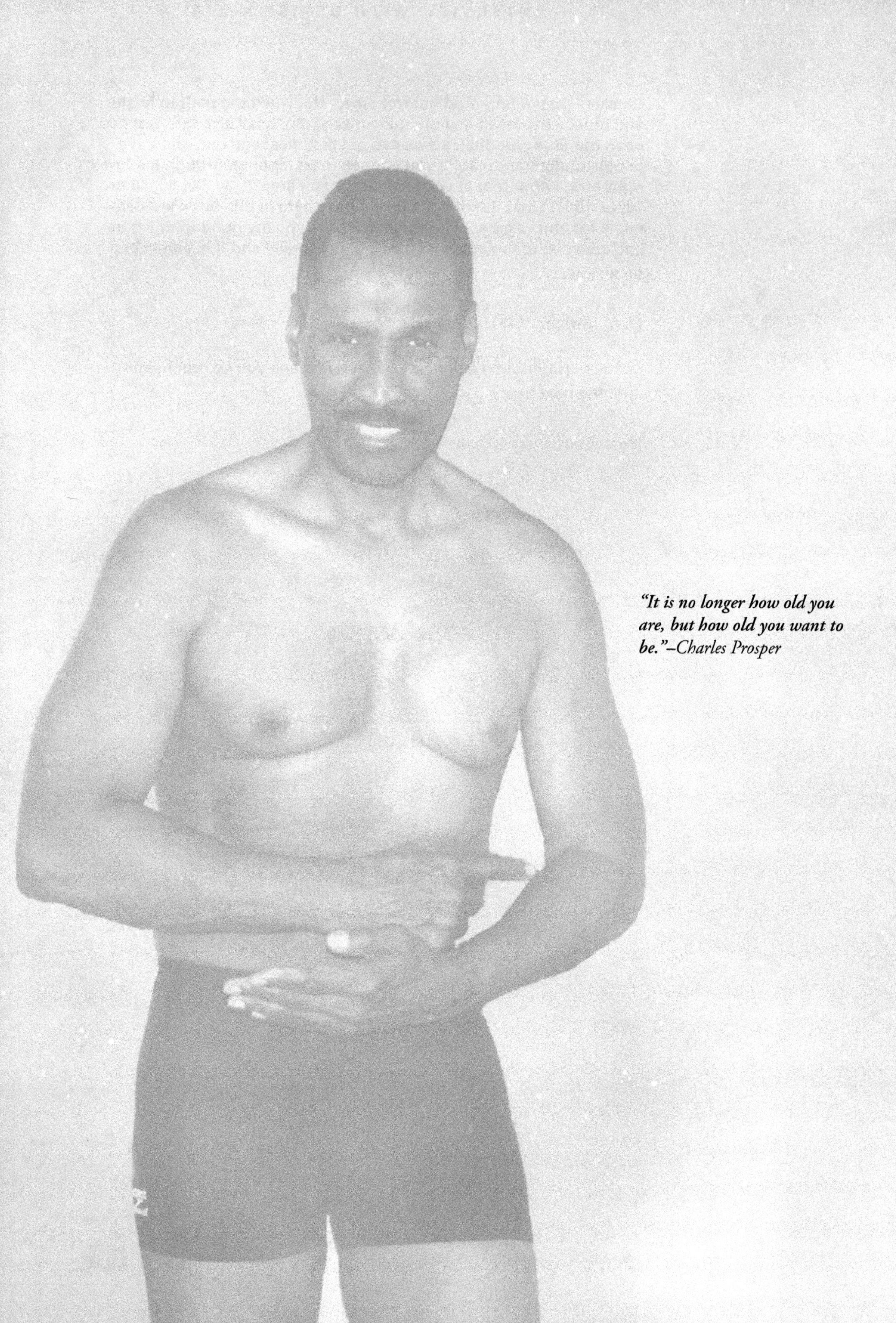

"It is no longer how old you are, but how old you want to be."–Charles Prosper

Why This Book Is For Men In Their 30's

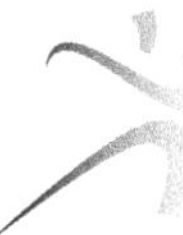

Jay Godfrey has been my neighbor and garden workout partner periodically for over 3 years. Here in this interview, he gives his insights as to why *"How To Get Fit Fast AT Any Age"* is for everyone, male or female, regardless of their age group.

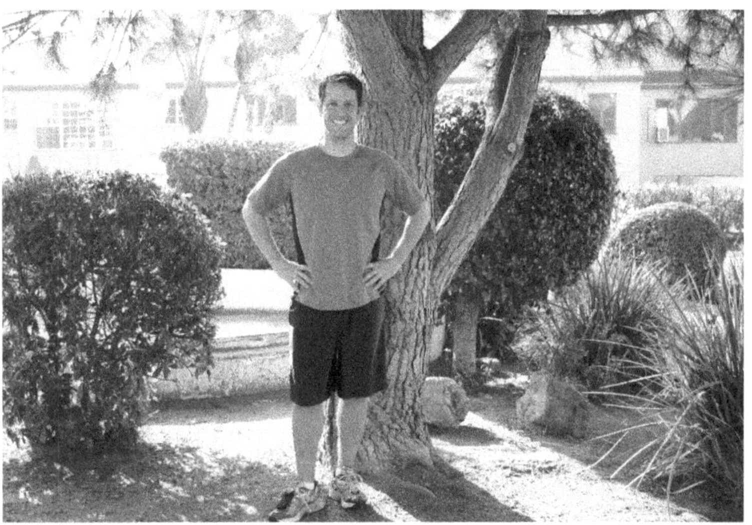

Jay Godfrey (Fit at 31)

Photography by Charles Prosper

Charles: **This is yours truly Charles Prosper. I'm here with my friend and my neighbor, Jay Godfrey, and workout buddy. We have been working out in the garden, oh, for a few years now, and I have given Jay some pointers. Jay pointed out something to me, after he read the book. He mentioned that, though the title of the book *"How To Get Fit Fast At Any Age"* is catchy, and means just that. Jay is 33 years old, and Jay was telling me that he's gotten quite a bit from the book, and from the principles of it, and he is just going to tell us today why he thinks that what's inside here is for any age group for a person who is serious in doing physical fitness. How're you doing today, Jay?**

Jay: Good. Good. Glad to be here. Glad to help you out with this project.

Charles: **Okay, and we're out here in the garden. We're in our work-out area today.**

Jay: We are. We're out here in the garden of iron. *(Laughter.)*

Charles: ***(Continued laughter.)*** **The garden of iron, that's it. Now, the thing we were talking about before is that people are so hung up on gyms and the age thing, so that makes them procrastinate and not want to take any action. So, you pointed out to me...How old are you, Jay?**

Jay: I'm 31 actually. You said 33, so I correct the record. *(Laughter.)*

Charles: **Okay, good to be corrected and on record. Now, you've read the book haven't you?**

Jay: Yeah. Yeah.

Charles: **And now, I want you to speak on behalf of those who are like, in their late 20's and early 30's...The book says how to get fit after fifty, and I've taken a little heat about the fact that it's not just a book about people over fifty. What would be your comment on that?**

"Nothing is secret because somebody knows it."– Luzemily Prosper (author's daughter at 10-years old)

Jay: Well, I think that you're right, what you said at the end there. It's not just a book for people over forty or fifty because the principles you got in this book are universal. I mean, good nutrition, getting out doing something every day – whether it would be hitting the weights, whether it would be doing a little cardio, those type of things – that's going to work for anybody! I mean, if you limit your calorie intake. If you can burn more calories that you can take in, through exercise, then you're going to lose weight. You're going to get fit. You're going to drop fat percentage off your body mass, and you're going to get in better shape. So, I think it's not just a book for people over fifty, over forty, over sixty, whatever age group you want to say. It's a book for anybody! Anybody can use it.

Charles: **Um hum. Because you've used these same principles with me out here for years, haven't you?**

Jay: Yeah, I have, and I've seen great results. And you know, I'm going to take another little angle on this, something that I've realized working with you is that you don't need to spend a lot of money. A few simple weights, used every day, will do the same trick as an expensive gym membership. So, you don't have to be super-complicated, just simple back-to-the-basics type stuff is going to benefit you. It's going to make you feel a lot better.

Charles: **And you know, that's amazing that you bring that up because that's the same thing that Denise Kenny said when I interviewed her. She pointed out that a lot of people don't want to go to professional gyms because, women especially, who are self-conscious of their weight, as they're walking in, don't want everybody looking at them. They don't want to have to wear the tight leotards. They don't want to feel like they are on the spot. They get stressed out when they have to go to the gym with all of the gorgeous bodies walking around them, and they feel like all of the eyes are on them. So, we've been working out with these simple weights here for years, and it's not complicated.**

Jay: Exactly. Exactly. And, you know, people are self-conscious, and you go to a gym, and it's more about how can you lift, and what do you look like, and all of those types of things whereas this book teaches us how to just simply workout in your basement, in your back yard...if you're lucky enough to live in a beautiful place like Southern California where it's good weather all time. *(Laughter.)*

Charles: **And we're in the garden of iron.**

"Life is not short if you spend it well."–Luzemily Prosper (author's daughter at 11-years old)

Jay: That's right. In January... *(Continued laughter.)* and it's beautiful weather, you don't need all that stuff. You need a little determination. You need a few simple things to help you out, but this book would work for anyone. And it's a healthy, safe way to do it. I mean, even a young high school student maybe trying to get in shape to go out for the football team, the basketball team or baseball team, could use these same principles because they're safe; they're healthy. You're not out advocating that we lift a lot of heavy weights or do anything crazy. Everything is safe. Everything is effective. This is a book for any age group. Anybody that wants to get in shape, wants to lose some weight, wants to feel better about themselves, and just feel better in general, these principles are going to work for them.

Charles: **Absolutely, and the thing that I just want to bring home and emphasize is the fact to simplify. I think the total investment in our outdoor in-the-garden gym has probably been no more than $250, $350 at max. And the thing about it, you don't have to get it all at once. You can just start with a bench and a barbell.**

Jay: Yep. Exactly.

Charles: **You don't have to start with all that fancy stuff. Then after a while, you get some dumbbells. After a while you get, say, a sit-up bench. After that, maybe you want to get some power stands. And then, you just work into it, but you start somewhere – because if you wait until everything is perfect, you wait until you have the time to go to the gym, or you want to wait until you can get the most expensive home gym – it's just going to be another reason to procrastinate. Wouldn't you agree?**

Jay: Oh, yeah. Absolutely. And you know, I think the idea of being simple is one of the things I learned the most from you. I remember a little while back, I was out here working out with you, and you just gave me a couple of tips. Maybe you want to drop your weight down a little bit on what you're lifting, and focus on your technique a little more. I've seen that pay huge dividends, just being a little more simple and take some of that machismo out of it, and just say, okay, I'm just going to focus on my technique of what I'm doing here with this lift and not worry so much about lifting huge amounts of weight. And doing like this out here simply and by yourself, you have to be a little more careful. You don't have someone spotting you all the time, but then you're not worried about, hey boy, if I don't lift x amount of weight then all of the other big muscle gargantuans in the gym...

Charles: ***(Laughter.)***

Jay: ...are going to be poking fun at me. *(Laughter.)* Whereas here if you do it simply on your own, that sort of thing, or maybe with a close family member, brother, spouse, girlfriend, boyfriend...

"If it was illegal to hug - nobody would be happy."– Luzemily Prosper (author's daughter at 10-years old)

Charles: **Or neighbor!**

Jay: Yeah, friend, neighbor, you don't have to worry so much about those things. You're more concerned about more, hey, I'm going to help you feeling better, getting into the best shape you can be in, and you're going to help me, and that's what the whole point of this is. That we feel good – every day.

Charles: **Absolutely, well that basically is the message that we're driving home here. And, Jay, I really, really appreciate your taking the time here...just before your workout actually...to give us this interview. And Jay, I want to help you out. I want to give you a little plug. Not many people know that you also are a model and actor. Is that so?**

Jay: That's right. Yeah. I focus a little more on the acting side than the modeling side due to the fact that I'm not over 6 feet tall. (Laughter.) That cuts out a lot of the modeling jobs.

Charles: **Well, if anybody wants to get in contact with Jay, for the modeling that you do, they can contact you through your Facebook page?**

Jay: Yeah. Yeah. Just search Jay Godfrey on Facebook, and they should find me. I'm located in Los Angeles, California.

Charles: **Okay. Pleasure again, my good friend. Thanks so much.**

Jay: Thank you.

Charles: **Hey, since we're out here, let's pump some iron.**

Jay: Sounds good to me. *(Laughter.)*

"When you do good things, good things happen."– *Luzemily Prosper (author's daughter at 10-years old)*

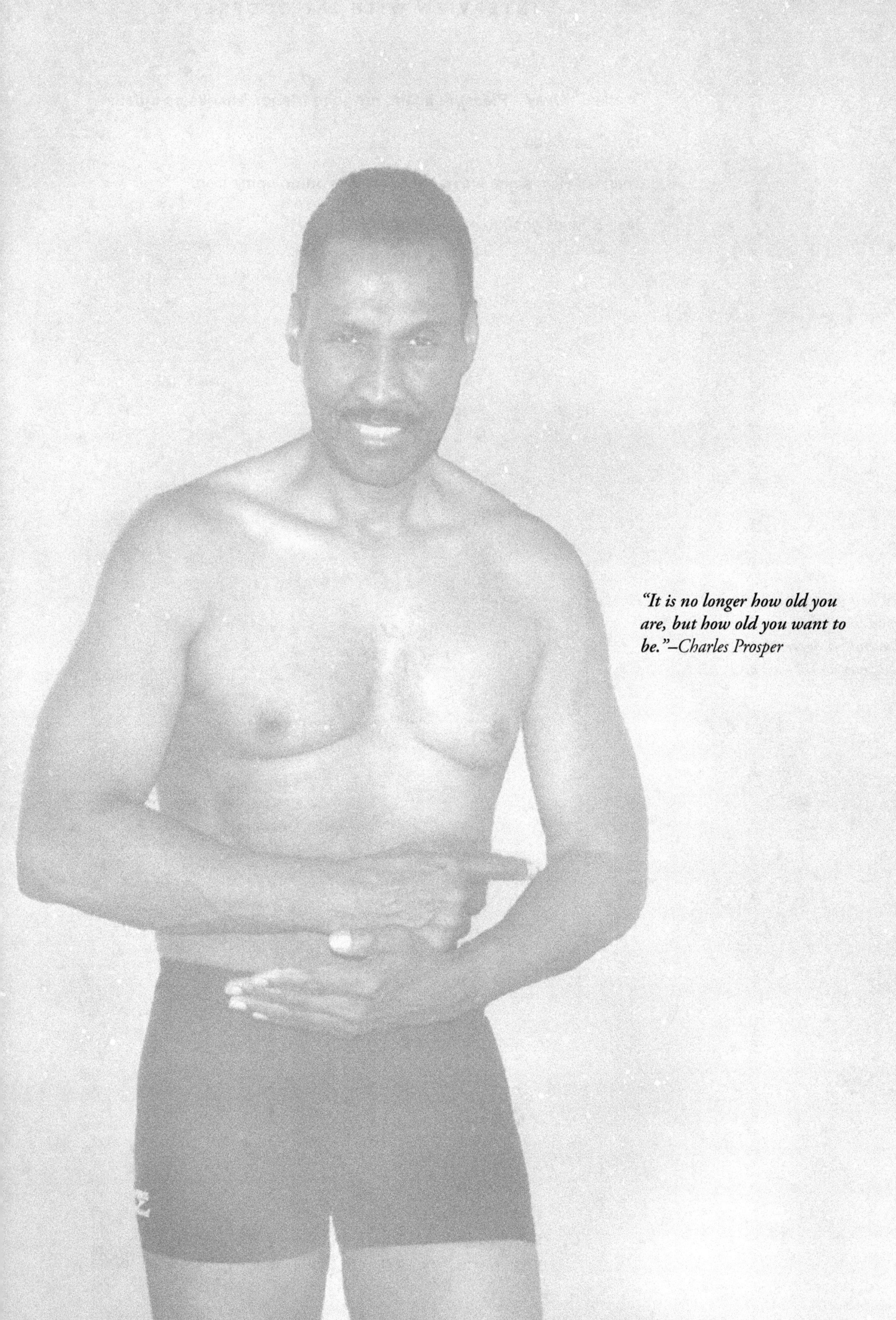

"It is no longer how old you are, but how old you want to be."–Charles Prosper

CHAPTER 16

Final Thoughts

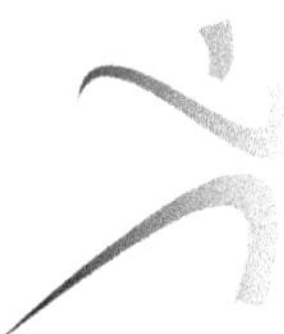

This is a book about and for those who want to make a positive change in their lives. I feel that if you are not alone and if others depend on you, it is not a luxury but a duty to take care of yourself. You just ain't gonna get another bod'. This is it. And if you were to just stop and take a moment to put yourself in the awe of the miracle of your human body, you might, you just might be inspired to take care of it and appreciate it more. Don't take your health for granted.

"I am at the stage of my life where I know that the majority of people will never do what the minority of successful people are <u>always</u> willing to do."–Charles Prosper

Books Up The Stairs

I had an experience once that made me see quite clearly, how blessed we all are to have a body with which we *can* improve. Let me tell you what happened to me one day while giving a business workshop at a local community college.

I regularly sold books at the end of each workshop, so I usually took with me several boxes, depending on the size of the class. The class was on the third floor, and I would usually just take the freight elevator to haul me and my cases of books, placed on a hand truck, up to my class. But on this bright and sunny afternoon day, the elevators were out of order...so, I had to place my boxes of books on my dolly, and pull them up three flights of stairs, step-by-step. I was fussing and fuming, mad and mumbling to myself at the incompetency of the college allowing the freight elevators to get out of order and not fixing them rapidly so impatient and fatigued professors like myself wouldn't have to haul them, huffing and puffing up the stairs. And I continue to bitch and moan about my plight, I finally made it up to the top landing of the class. Just at that very moment, a young man, quadriplegic, paralyzed from the neck down, driving his motorized wheelchair with slight right and left movements of his neck, rolls right in front of me and says with a smile: "Beautiful day for a walk, isn't it." Wow! I almost started crying, right then and there with the realization of how blessed I truly was to have all of my limbs with the ability to have pulled those books up those stairs. Do you think that quadriplegic young man would have minded trading places with me in order to be able to experience what it feels like to pull several boxes up three flights of stairs by his own effort? Yes, ladies and gentlemen, each of you are truly blessed.

Sometimes we just need a wake up call to allow us to see it. Now, if you don't take action and just let your body continue to deteriorate, that indeed is your prerogative. I most surely will not stop talking to you because you refuse to take care of yourself, but my question to you is, if this is the case, why? Isn't health and happiness the end of every activity that we do? Some people, because of certain physical handicaps or diseases, can't do anything to improve their physical condition. But if *you* can, I ask you again, why not?

Why Exercise? The Swamp vs. Flowing Spring Waters

I want you to think about something for a moment. I want you to think of a swamp. Okay. Got that image in your mind? Now, I want you to think of flowing mountain spring waters. Got *that* image in mind? Could you describe the differences in the two? Let us first take the swamp. A swamp is characterized by stagnation, filth and putrefaction. Not all organisms are turned off by the idea of living in the habitat of a swamp. Fungi and moss love it there - so do frogs, snakes and lizards - and flies. It smells bad, and it is slimy to walk through.

Now, what are the characteristics of flowing mountain spring waters? For one, it's clean enough to drink, but the essence and the secret of its purity lies in the fact that it *flows*. It moves and circulates, and in a way, keeps itself clean from the accumulation of filth and sediment.

"Don't be afraid to take a big step if one is indicated. You can't cross a chasm in two small jumps."–David Lloyd George

Using this as a metaphor of the difference of one who exercises and one who doesn't, we can see the parallel and what essentially happens to us as we age and become sedentary, stagnate and deteriorating through inactivity. Just like the sedentary swamp, we begin to accumulate all of the filth, sediment and putrefaction of not using our bodies.

Now, what would happen to the swamp that begun to flow? What would happen to the waters that would begin to move and circulate through the rocks and down the mountain edges? Yes, all of the sediment and filth would begin to purify itself from the waters. Beginning and continuing with regular physical exercise, no matter at what stage of your life, will in turn, reverse the physiological deterioration of the aging process. With exercise and proper eating, the living waters of your blood, heart and circulatory system, begin to rejuvenate your body, giving it new life and new energy.

Beginning to exercise must be taken and understood to be the beginning of a new lifestyle. You are not doing this to get somewhere - then stop. No more do you bathe today - to become clean enough to stop bathing for the rest of your life. There are undeniable daily activities that must be done for the rest of our lives. Some of them are more obvious like eating, sleeping, bathing. I say that exercising also belongs on this list, that is, if you want to live longer, feel stronger and enjoy more of your life. Why not give yourself a chance to experience more of life? I encourage you to begin and take that first step, and I stand up and applaud you for honoring your body, for to do this is to honor the temple of your spirit.

"Success usually comes to those who are too busy to be looking for it."–Henry David Thoreau

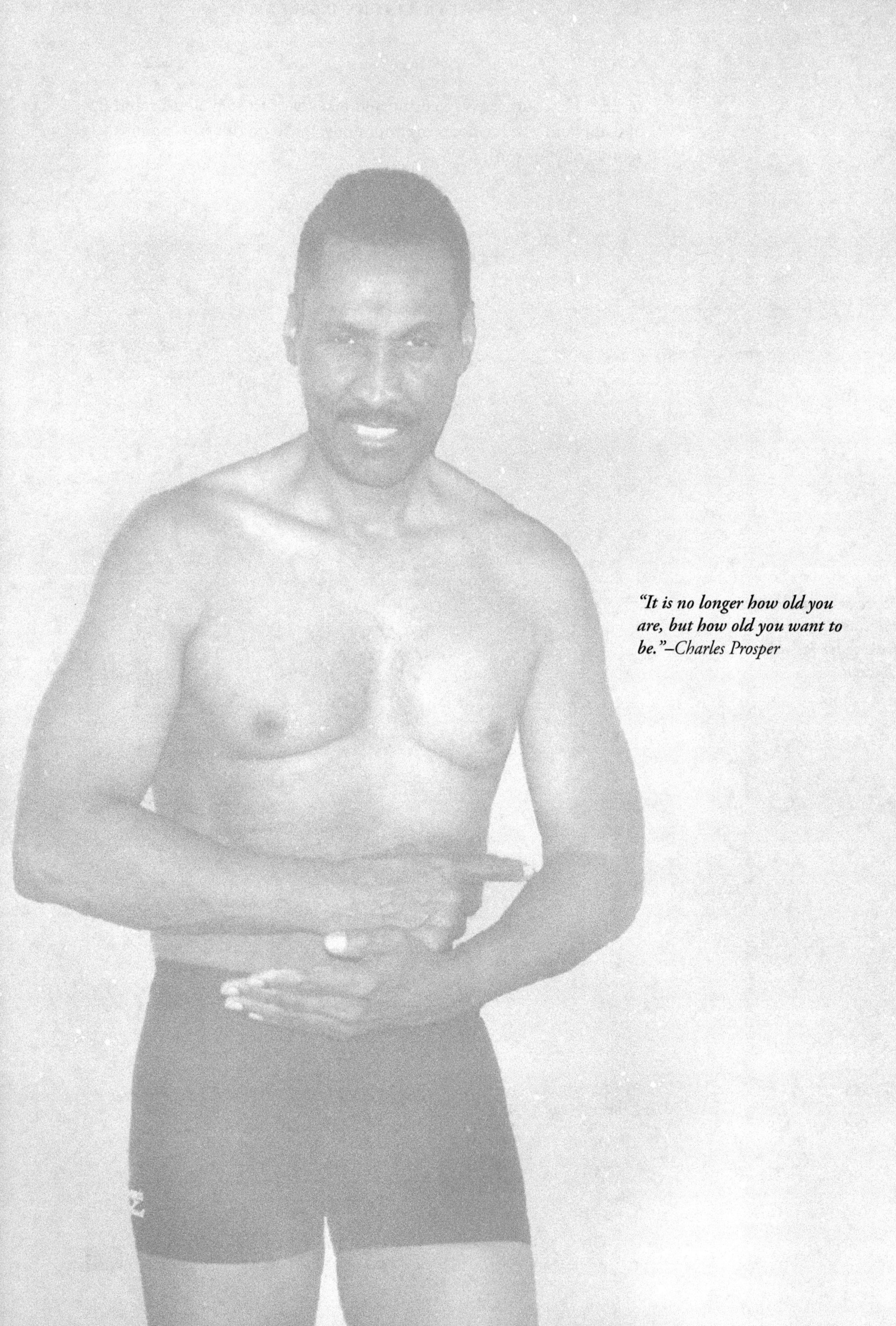

"It is no longer how old you are, but how old you want to be."–Charles Prosper

17 CHAPTER

Are You Ready To Take The Next Step?

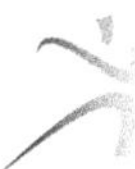

"Though no one can go back and make a brand new start, ANYONE can start from now and make a brand new ending."–Anonymous

Look, I know how hard it can be to get started. Let me personally help you. Allow me to be your personal 12-Week Fit Fast fitness coach. No matter what shape you are in, no matter where

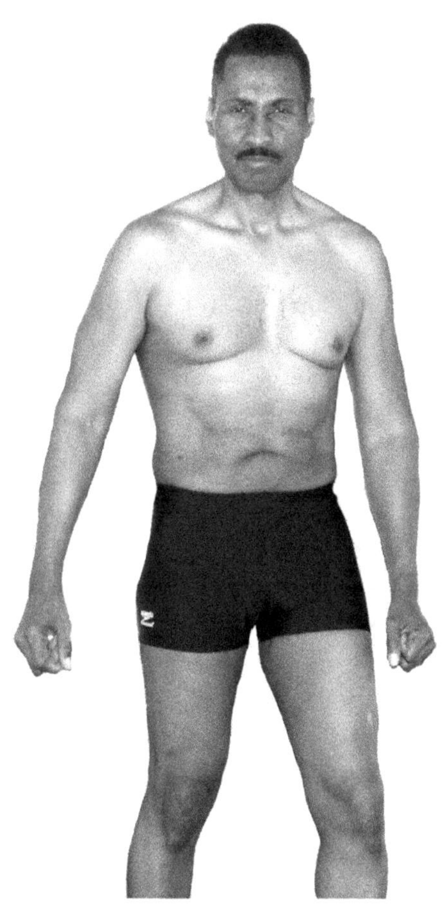

Charles Prosper (Your Personal Fitness Coach)

you are in the world, I can help you with a personalized fitness coaching program. I want to show you off in the next edition of this book which will feature real life before and after success stories. You can download your FREE 12-Week eCourse right now. Just go to:

www.FitFastAtAnyAge.com

All the best, *Charles Prosper*

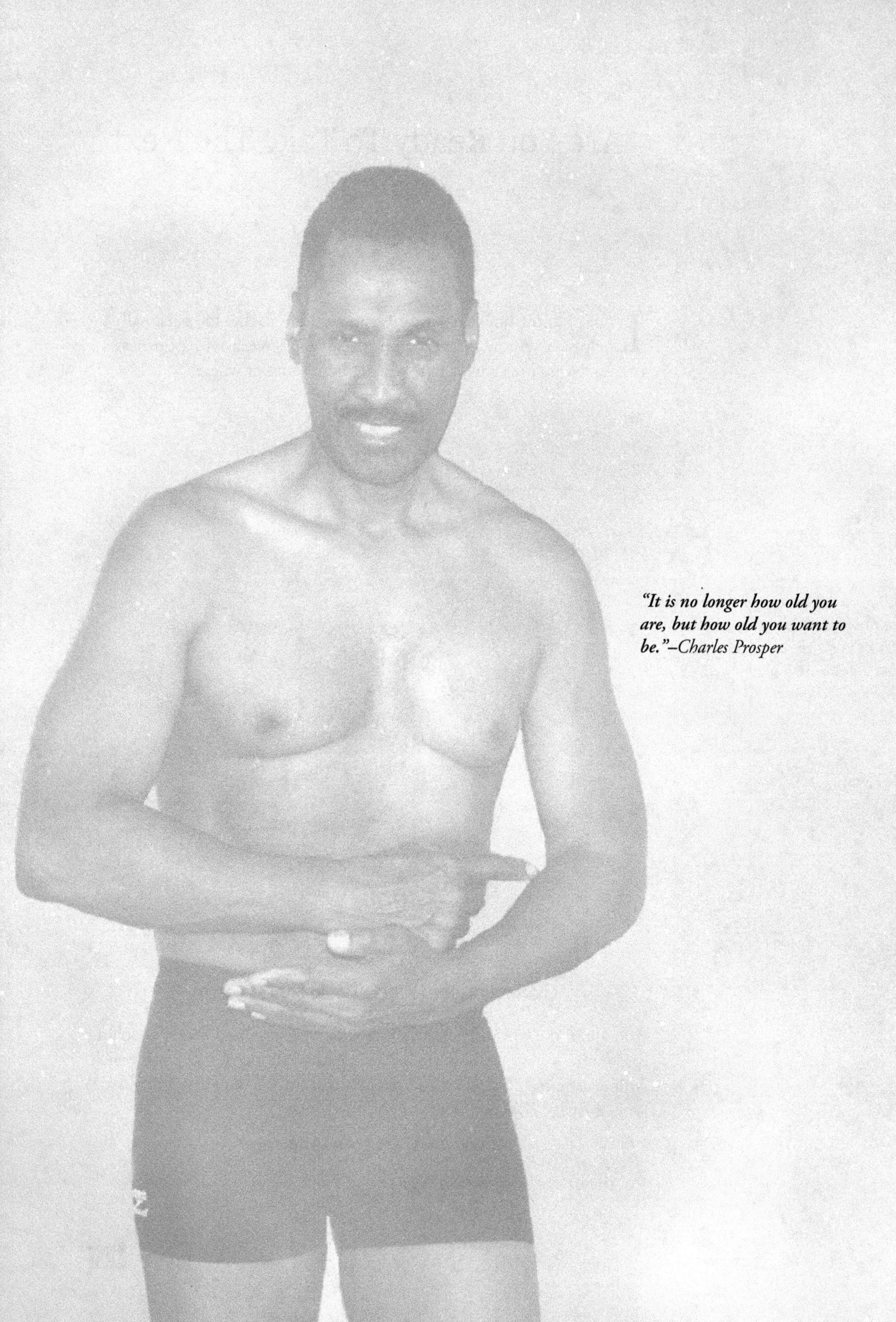

"It is no longer how old you are, but how old you want to be."–Charles Prosper

CHAPTER 18

About The Author

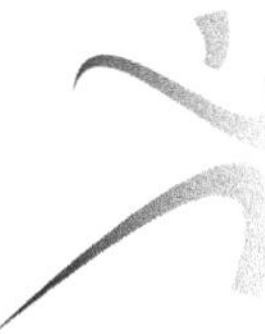

Charles Prosper is no stranger to books on self-help, success, sports and personal development. He is an author of over 7 books on these topics, two of his most recent books include The Secret Revealed, How To Use The 12 Great Laws of Success (ISBN-10 0-943845-46-7), as well as Fighting Secrets of Martial Arts Masters (ISBN-978-0943845-29-6) both published by Global Publishing Company of Los Angeles, California, and available on Amazon.com.

Charles is dedicated to being a vanguard in the field of self-betterment and personal growth.

"God's ear lies close to the believer's lip."–Anonymous

Charles Prosper Is Available for All Interviews

Need an expert interview on health, fitness or nutrition? Contact Charles today.

Charles Prosper Is Available To Speak for Your Group or Organization

Need a captivating speaker on health, fitness or nutrition? Contact Charles today.

How To Attend A Live Charles Prosper *Fit Fast* Workshop

See here the latest schedule of all of the live Charles Prosper *Fit Fast* Workshops held in Southern California and other parts of the country:

http://www.ProsperWorkshops.com

You can always contact Charles by going to his website:

www.FitFastAtAnyAge.com

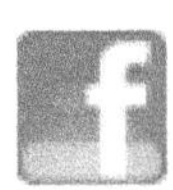

Become a friend on **Facebook**

http://www.facebook.com/cprosper?ref=name

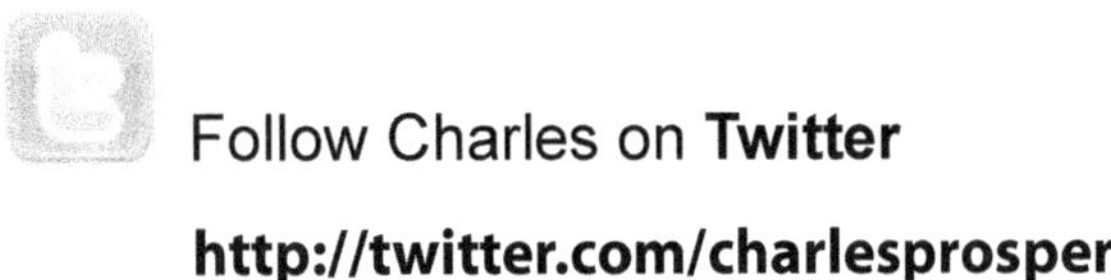

Follow Charles on **Twitter**

http://twitter.com/charlesprosper

Recommended Reading

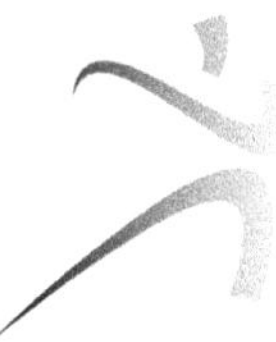

If this book makes me look tall, it is because I stand on the shoulders of giants. I highly recommend that you also read these great books, on health and exercise, that will move you exponentially to your ultimate fitness success.

The Lean Body Promise, Lee Labrada. ISBN 0-06-059371-7 $24.95

Body For Life, Bill Phillips. ISBN 0-06-019339-5 $26.95

The Calorie King® – Fat & Carbohydrate Counter, Allan Borushek. ISBN 978-1-930448-29-2 $12.99

Strength Training Anatomy, Frédéric Delavier. ISBN 0-7360-4185-0 $18.95

"Peace is not the same as happiness because peace has no opposite. You can be happy or sad and still be peaceful." *– Luzemily Prosper (author's daughter at 10-years old)*

www.ingramcontent.com/pod-product-compliance
Lightning Source LLC
LaVergne TN
LVHW061241100826
845148LV00008B/1007